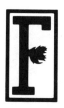

House Calls

GERALD COUZENS

A FIRESIDE BOOK
Published by
SIMON & SCHUSTER
New York   London   Toronto   Sydney   Tokyo   Singapore

FIRESIDE

Simon & Schuster Building
Rockefeller Center
1230 Avenue of the Americas
New York, New York, 10020

FIRESIDE and colophon are registered trademarks
of Simon & Schuster Inc.

Illustrations by Arleen Frasca
Designed by Quinn Hall
Manufactured in the United States of America

10   9   8   7   6   5   4   3   2   1

Library of Congress Cataloging in Publication Data
Housecalls : how doctors treat themselves and their
own families for common illnesses and injuries /
[edited by] Gerald Couzens.
        p.   cm.
    "A Fireside book."
    Includes index.
    1. Medicine, Popular.   I. Couzens, Gerald.
II. Title: House calls.
RC81.H873   1993
610—dc20   92-41246
                                      CIP

ISBN: 0-671-76740-2

The ideas, procedures, and suggestions in this book
are intended to supplement, not replace, the medical
advice of trained professionals. In addition, all matters
regarding your health require medical supervision.
Consult your physician before adopting the medical
suggestions in this book, as well as about any
condition that may require diagnosis or medical
attention.

The authors and publishers disclaim any liability
arising directly or indirectly from the use of this book.

Contents

THE FEET

SKIN AND HAIR

GENERAL PROBLEMS

APPENDICES

Introduction

HOW TO USE THIS BOOK

*H*ouse Calls might be called "How Physicians Heal Themselves." Its purpose is to provide to you the inside information that physicians use to treat themselves for their own minor, everyday medical problems.

More than eighty leading physicians and medical specialists provide this much-valued information in their own words. One of the reasons these doctors are all leaders in their field is that they are uniformly excellent communicators, who not only cut through all the medical jargon but possess that rarest of medical skills—empathy. They give advice for the most common medical problems we encounter— from athlete's foot to dandruff—literally from head to toe. It's like having your own private consultation with one of the leading experts in his or her field. In easy-to-understand language, learn what a leading sports medicine specialist does to alleviate ankle sprains and tendinitis. Listen while a top dermatologist tells you how best to treat sunburn with a proved home remedy, or an allergist tells you his secrets for combating hay fever. This book also provides a wealth of prevention tips to avoid many of these minor—but very annoying—ailments.

The doctors also help guide you through the labyrinth of over-the-counter (OTC) medications available for just about any minor medical problem. This inside tour of your pharmacist's shelves offers advice as to which ingredients to look for in OTC medications, and why. The doctors also tell you which specific brand names they believe are most effective. They also warn against OTC products which are ineffective—and sometimes harmful—despite the advertising claims made for them.

In addition, the doctors offer medical guidance as to when a seemingly "minor" medical problem may be a signal of a more serious one. This guide appears under the heading "Cause for Concern" in each ailment section. To offer further guidance, at the beginning of each chapter, some important medical problems and symptoms are listed, which the experts say require the attention of a medical doctor.

By providing this assistance, the book can help you develop a greater sense of your own health. You will learn to take a logical approach to minor medical problems and know when something needs immediate medical attention. And, by becoming better informed and understanding all you can about your ailment, your visit with your physician will be more productive.

As complete as *House Calls* is for treating everyday medical ailments, bear in mind that it is not meant to be a substitute for your doctor. Nor is it intended to be a guide for self-diagnosis. Also bear in mind that the practice of medicine is as much art as science, and different doctors may hold different opinions regarding the treatment of the same illness. In a few cases, some of the doctors in this book even have different views about treatment alternatives. Most important, if any information in this book conflicts with what your physician tells you, follow your physician's advice.

The medical experts also warn that any physical symptom—no matter how minor it may appear—should not be ignored or considered unimportant. In particular, any symptom that persists, or recurs, should be brought to the attention of your physician. This is especially true if you've never experienced the symptom before. For example, if you've long suffered from a periodic "sour" stomach—and your physician does not consider it a serious medical problem —then this symptom may not be as significant for you as it would be for someone who experiences it for the first time. Always listen to your body, and when you sense something is not right, consult your physician. In almost every medical problem, the sooner it is diagnosed, the more likely it can be cured.

The Eyes

GENERAL INFORMATION

The eyes are complex, delicate, and extremely sensitive tissues that receive and transmit vast amounts of information to the brain each minute. Of the five senses, sight is by far the most important, as it is estimated that 80 percent of our acquired knowledge comes from processing visual stimuli. Protecting the eyes, therefore, is obviously vitally important.

Here's how the eyes "see": light first enters the eye through the cornea—the transparent dome covering the front of the eyeball—traveling from there through the aqueous humor, the watery anterior area that is located behind the cornea and in front of the lens. It then passes through the lens of the eye and into the vitreous humor, the jellylike substance that fills the

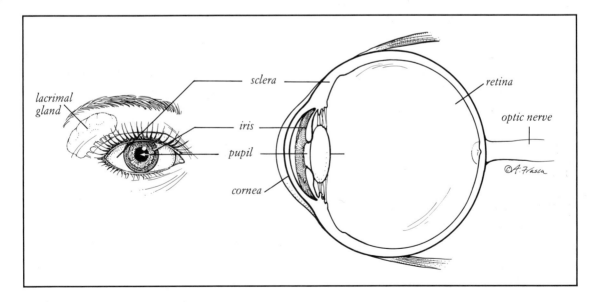

eye behind the lens, and is received by the light sensitive cells (rods and cones) of the retina in the interior of the eye. The brain receives light impulses via the optic nerve, and we're able to see what we're looking at.

The eyes continuously adapt to changes in light. According to some studies, harsh light and continued exposure to the sun's ultraviolet rays can cause eye redness and dryness, and over a period of years may lead to cataracts, a more serious condition typified by a clouding of the lens in the eye.

The eyes self-lubricate with tears from the conjunctiva, the thin lining of the eyeball and eyelid, and the lacrimal glands located above each eyeball. The tears not only clean the eye but help kill any bacteria that develop on the visible parts of the eye or the eyelids. Common problems triggered by bacteria and viruses include blepharitis, styes, and conjunctivitis, a contagious variety of which is known as pink eye, and ulcers of the cornea.

The eyes are supported and protected from impact injury by the orbit, the circular "socket" made up of bone from the cheek, eyebrow, and nose. The eyelids form another protective screen for the eyes. They keep out foreign bodies and shield the eyes from harmful light and scratches. The conjunctiva, the moist, transparent mucus membrane that covers the inner part of the eyelids and white part of the eyes, also protects the eyes, makes tears, and ensures the smooth movement of the lids when blinking.

EYE EMERGENCIES

CHEMICAL BURNS. Caustic chemicals splashed in the eye can cause permanent damage. To treat, immediately pull the eyelid back, keeping the eye wide open. Flush the eye with water from a faucet or container for up to 30 minutes. Contact ophthalmologist or go directly to hospital Emergency Department.

SCRATCHED CORNEA. Acute eye pain, swelling, and redness occur whenever the cornea is scratched by a sharp object. Keep the eye closed or cover it with a patch. Contact ophthalmologist or go to the hospital Emergency Department.

DETACHED RETINA. Trauma, aging, or underlying disease causes the retina to tear and then painlessly peel away from its blood supply. Symptoms include flashing, jagged lights; blurred vision; or shadows moving across the eye. Contact ophthalmologist for treatment.

PHYSICIAN'S CARE REQUIRED

GLAUCOMA. Increased pressure within the eyeball that can lead to blindness. Chronic glaucoma develops over time and strikes without warning. Acute glaucoma, a rare form, often manifests itself with blurred vision or halos around lights and objects. Glaucoma cannot be prevented but can be treated with surgery.

CATARACTS. This clouding of the eye lens can accompany aging, but may be caused by diabetes or prolonged use of corticosteroid drugs. Symptoms include blurred vision, impaired night vision, and halos that appear around lights and objects. Correctable by surgery.

COMMON EYE PROBLEMS

BLACK EYE
Discoloration of the skin surrounding the eyes and often a reddening of the white of the eye. Caused by a sharp blow to the eye, forehead, nose, or even the scalp. *Requires* medical attention. **Page 14**

DRY EYE
Brought on by arid climates, rheumatoid arthritis, insufficient tear production, eyelid abnormalities, surface infections, aging, or as a reaction to certain cosmetics or medications. Major symptoms are eye redness, a hot, sandy sensation in the eyes, and, often, continuous tearing-up. **Page 17**

EYE REDNESS
On awakening, the sclera, or white portion of the eye, appears red, and eyes feel warm if the lids are closed. Causes include heat; contact lenses; allergic reaction; conjunctivitis; injury; hot, dry climates. **Page 16**

FLASHES/FLOATERS
Flashes appear as flashing lights or bolts of lightning though no external light source is present. Quite common as people age. Floaters are small specks that appear to be moving through the field of vision. **Page 19**

FOREIGN BODIES
Any tiny foreign object on the surface of the eye that brings on pain. **Page 12**

PINK EYE
Inflammation of the conjunctiva, the membrane that covers both the eyelid and the eyeball. Symptoms include a pink or red tinge to the whites of the eyes and swollen eyelids. **Page 21**

STYE
A sore, red bump on the eyelid often caused by infection in the eyelash follicle. **Page 23**

EYE CARE SPECIALISTS

OPHTHALMOLOGIST (M.D.). An ophthalmologist is a physician and surgeon who has at least four years of intensive training after medical school and specializes in eye care. An ophthalmologist treats all eye disorders, screens for glaucoma, gives vision testing, prescribes lenses for eyeglasses and contacts, prescribes medicine, and performs surgery and laser treatments.

OPTOMETRIST (O.D.). An optometrist is not a medical doctor, but studies for four years at an optometric college. He offers vision testing, screens for glaucoma, prescribes and fits both eyeglass lenses and contact lenses. Optometrists can treat external eye diseases in some states, and prescribe medication. They cannot perform eye surgery or laser treatment.

OPTICIAN. An optician is licensed by the state to fill prescriptions for eyeglasses and contact lenses.

BLACK EYE

James C. Newton, M.D.

Dr. Newton is the director of Ophthalmology, St. Luke's/Roosevelt Hospital Center in New York

A black eye can be rather dramatic looking, but it often looks worse than it actually is. The vivid colors associated with this impact injury develop after several hours, and it can be two weeks before the black, greenish, and yellow of the "shiner" finally disappear completely from the eye area. (Cosmetic concerns should be the least of your worries when you get hit in the eye, however.)

Treatment

Whenever you're struck in the eye, whether while playing sports or accidentally running into or being hit by something, you need to be examined by an ophthalmologist as soon as possible. In the interim, the only effective self-care is to close the eye and apply an ice pack directly over it. Use a cold can of soda if you don't have ice. The cold temperature keeps swelling to a minimum. If the eye is swollen shut, there's nothing a doctor can do—exclusive of expensive sonograms, MRIs, and CT scans—until the swelling eventually goes down.

By immediately combating the swelling, you are also reducing the level of internal bleeding, which causes the black and blue discoloration of the eye.

Do not take aspirin for pain relief. Aspirin thins the blood and prevents it from clotting. Instead, take two acetaminophen (Tylenol) tablets. This should provide some pain relief and won't encourage further bleeding.

Cause for Concern

Double vision, or an inward turning of your eye when you look straight ahead, is a sign that you may have suffered a "blow-out" fracture. This is a cracking of the thin bone serving as the floor and wall of the orbit of your eye. Surgery may be necessary.

Blurry vision can be expected with a blow to the eye and must be evaluated by an ophthalmologist. Fortunately, most blurred vision clears as swelling decreases.

What the Doctor Will Do

A complete eye examination after injury must include the following: a careful vision test; a check for ocular motility (ability to move) to rule out blowout fractures of the orbit; a careful slit-lamp examination (that intense light projected into the eye); and an ophthalmoscopic examination. Any visual change resulting from injury must be carefully evaluated.

The slit-lamp examination enables the doctor to examine the surface and anterior portion of the eye. The cornea is evaluated for abrasions and the anterior chamber for internal inflammatory signs (iritis). The lens of the eye is examined to make sure there are no movements signifying dislocation.

Ocular pressure is tested as well, because getting hit may recess the drainage angle, resulting in secondary glaucoma. There may also be a rupture of the globe not visible because of bleeding and location, resulting in a condition known as soft eye.

In the ophthalmoscopic examination the doctor will most importantly check the back of the eye for any trouble with the retina. He will note swelling and bleeding, but primarily check for retinal damage and/or retinal detachment. When a retinal tear is discovered immediately after it occurs, it usually requires minimal treatment and has a very high success rate.

Undiscovered retinal tears often lead to retinal detachments, necessitating more involved treatments. If a tear in the retina is not properly diagnosed at the time of the accident, the patient risks loss of his or her eyesight or may suffer extensive surgery to repair a retinal detachment.

I cannot stress how very important it is to be checked for these tears. I've seen cases, where, because they were not uncovered at the time of initial injury, or shortly thereafter, the tears turned to complete retinal detachments and serious consequences.

Prevention

- Wear protective eyewear for sports and potentially hazardous activity.
- Make sure lenses on goggles are made of polycarbonate, a plastic that is 100 times stronger than glass, resists shattering, and also softens impact.
- For low impact sports, such as volleyball, the lenses should be 2 mm thick, whereas for basketball, racket sports, and baseball, lenses should be at least 3 mm thick.
- Make sure the eyewear has a padded nose bridge for shock absorption and additional comfort.
- Wear an adjustable head strap to ensure good fit.

WHAT TO DO

- Apply an ice pack or cold can of soda over the closed eye to reduce swelling.

- Take acetaminophen (Tylenol) for pain relief.
- Call your physician.

EYE REDNESS

Robert H. Meaders, M.D.

Dr. Meaders is the retina specialist for the Southwestern Eye Center, in Mesa, Arizona

Eye redness is often Mother Nature's warning that you need to give your eyes attention. Although you may think your problem is merely cosmetic, eye redness is never quite as simple as you imagine. It often requires either home treatment or a doctor's care.

Many of the conditions that cause the conjunctiva, the white outer covering of the eye, to redden can be treated successfully at home.

When both eyes are red, lack of sleep is often the cause. Eyes must replenish the epithelial cells that cover the cornea, and this is best done when the eyes are closed for extended periods during sleep. Neglect sleep, and the eyes become slightly pitted as the epithelial cells fall off and aren't replaced. Once the upper lid slides across this pitted surface, the blood vessels dilate and a reflex irritation develops, which results in red eyes.

Treatment

For people who have been awake all night and don't want to look red-eyed in the morning, 1–2 drops of commercially prepared eye drops will shrink the blood vessels in the eye and may cause the redness to disappear temporarily. But beware: when the medication wears off in an hour or so, the vessels will dilate abnormally, and the eyes will be as red or even redder than before.

For this reason, I don't recommend the use of astringent drops routinely, and I tell all my patients to stay away from any product that promises to get the red out of your eye. You want to put the moisture back into the eyes, not take out the red. Therefore, any OTC product that promotes itself as an artificial tear or ocular lubricant will do this best.

Artificial teardrops contain no medication and are simply a bland soothing saline solution containing appropriate amounts of potassium, calcium, and sundry micronutrients that mimic the tear film of your eyes. Artificial tears used regularly three or four times a day will make gritty, grimy eyes feel much better because the drops fill in the pitted eye surface and allow the upper lid to glide smoothly when you blink.

When you wear contact lenses too long,

eye redness is quite common because the epithelial cells that cover the clear window of the cornea begin to die off from lack of oxygen. As these cells fall from the eye, little nerves underneath are exposed, and this irritation quickly turns the eye red. When this occurs, the eyes will feel sore, as if you have sand in your eye.

To relieve this redness, don't wear your lenses for twelve to fourteen hours. Fresh air, along with sleep, will rapidly heal the eyes. If the redness does not disappear within twelve to twenty-four hours, see your eye specialist immediately.

Dry Eye

Dry eye, caused by too much sun exposure, wind, and low humidity will also cause eye redness. In arid parts of the country, many people develop dry-eye problems because the normal lubricating tears of the eyes evaporate quickly in the heat. Eyes can become so dry that they actually begin to crack like the desert floor. Once the condition becomes this serious, the emergency tear system comes on and intermittently floods the eyes as a protective device. This tearing leads people to mistaken their condition for "wet eye," but, in reality, dry eye is the problem.

Treatment

There is no permanent cure for dry eyes. To prevent the condition from developing, use OTC artificial teardrops on a regular basis. In some cases, this may mean 2 drops three to four times daily. If there are times when you don't have access to the drops, soak your closed eyes with a cool, wet facecloth for three to five minutes. This

helps constrict the blood vessels of the eye, and closing the eyes for this short time allows them to self-lubricate.

Another way to decrease chronic eye irritation and other damaging affects of the sun is to wear sunglasses that offer UV-A and UV-B protection when you are going to be outside for extended periods. If you wear clear prescription glasses for vision correction, have the lenses treated with special ultraviolet tinting or clear film to keep the sun's harmful rays from abusing your eyes.

Blepharitis

Blepharitis (or "granulated lids") is another ailment that causes eye redness. This minor eyelash infection usually affects people who have thin skin, fair hair, and pale complexions. The problem develops at the base of the eyelash and common symptoms include yellow, crusted, and matted eyelids, and eye redness.

Think of your eyelash follicles as missile silos. Each eyelash grows out of a separate hair "silo," or follicle, but when the follicle is overly large, the lash sits in it loosely, and bacteria enter easily. Infection soon develops, and pus oozes out along the eyelash, where it dries, crusts, and falls into the eye, causing chronic red eyes.

Treatment

Treatment for blepharitis is simple. Take a hot, damp facecloth and place it over the closed eyes for 5 minutes to soften the dry crust. Then, to remove all traces of this crust, take the washcloth and simply scrub back and forth across the closed eyelids like a child rubbing sleep out of his eyes.

Repeat this procedure when you wake up, at midday when the pus and oils accumulate, and then again at bedtime. Keeping the eyelids clean will take care of many cases without having to resort to antibiotics. The time blepharitis takes to clear up altogether varies among individuals.

What the Doctor Will Do

Vigilant eye hygiene may prevent blepharitis in those prone to it. However, if your case is persistent, your ophthalmologist will prescribe erythromycin or other antibiotic ointments to counteract the bacteria. After going through the cleaning routine with the warm washcloth, massage the ointment into the eyelashes in a gentle side-to-side motion, similar to that used to dislodge the crusts. This deposits the ointment around the base of the lash follicles and arrests the infection. Blepharitis tends to be a chronic condition and may require treatment indefinitely.

Cause for Concern

There's an old saying in ophthalmology: Beware of the patient with one red eye. Redness in only one eye typically means trouble, and a doctor's visit is usually in order. If redness appears in only one eye, if there is a history of glaucoma in your family, or if you've been working with metal or welding equipment and redness develops, contact your ophthalmologist. If you have allergies, take your medication or consult with your allergy specialist. Whenever your eye becomes red or painful and associated with vision loss or "foggy" vision, you should be seen immediately by an ophthalmologist.

To find out the cause of your one red eye, it's important first to review events of the day. Eye redness can easily be triggered by watching someone use welding equipment, for example, by standing close to someone who is grinding metal, or by bursting a superficial blood vessel in the conjunctiva of the eye. Also, if you're a contact lens wearer, the lens may be torn or something caught under the lens may be scratching the cornea.

Glaucoma, a serious eye disease brought on by abnormally high pressure in the eye, can also present itself with eye redness. If you develop eye redness and either you or someone in your family has glaucoma, this could be a warning sign of elevated eye pressure. Contact your ophthalmologist.

When checking in the mirror for the red, contact lens wearers should also be on the lookout for a white spot, a more serious condition that may develop on the cornea, the transparent, circular part of the front of the eyeball. A little white spot on the cornea means a corneal ulcer. Amoebic organisms that develop in homemade saltine solutions are the most serious cause, and if left unchecked, the amoeba will bore right through the cornea, and possibly lead to blindness.

To avoid corneal ulcers, only use commercially prepared saline solutions and follow the label directions carefully. Also, if you wear extended-wear lenses, clean them regularly and consult with your ophthalmologist when you have any signs of discomfort. The best lenses are the disposable variety that are worn for no more than the suggested five to seven days.

WHAT TO DO

- Maintain regular sleep hours.
- Put a cool, damp facecloth across your closed eyes to help constrict the blood vessels.
- Use artificial tears to help relieve the gritty feeling in the eyes and restore moisture.
- Do not use any OTC eye products that guarantee to "get the red out."
- Don't wear your contact lenses for twelve to fourteen hours after redness develops.
- In arid climates, lubricate the eyes several times daily with artificial teardrops.
- Wear UV-A and UV-B-protection sunglasses. Have your prescription glasses tinted with an ultraviolet coating to prevent sun damage.
- For blepharitis, place a hot, damp facecloth over closed eyes for 5 minutes. Then rub the cloth over the eyelids to remove the softened crusts.

FLASHES AND FLOATERS

W. Banks Anderson, M.D.

Dr. Anderson is professor of Ophthalmology at the Duke University Eye Center in Durham, North Carolina

Flashes

Many people who get hit in the eye say they see "stars." Actually, the flashing, often brilliant streaks of light they notice, have nothing to do with galactic sightings but are caused by the mechanical stimulation of the retina, the light-sensing inner layer of the eye.

Migraine sufferers (see HEADACHE, page 219) are well aware of seeing lights that are not there. In a classical case they suddenly see, off to one side, in both eyes, flickering, jagged lights and "heat waves." After 15–30 minutes the lights go away, but a pounding headache may follow.

If you're myopic (nearsighted) or have had any inflammation or injury to the eye, flashes can begin at an early age. But most causes of flashes are spontaneous and linked directly to the aging process. Between the ages of forty and sixty, flashes will randomly appear for no apparent reason. The gel inside the eye starts to liquefy and peel off from the retina. The tugging and pulling that goes on causes the retina to be stimulated, and the ensuing flashing, lightning streaks, and stars may continue on and off for several weeks until a layer of gel is stripped away.

Over 90 percent of the time this is a benign event related to aging and not associated with anything that produces long-term problems.

Cause for Concern

Every once in a while vitreous gel becomes stuck to the retina and tears it as it pulls away, and this needs to be treated because the tears are often precursors to retinal detachments.

Retinal tears are treated successfully in the doctor's office with either a laser or cryotherapy device. When your retina is detached, however, you will notice a shadow off to the side of your line of vision that begins to advance toward your line of sight. Hospitalization and surgery are required to repair a detached retina, and unfortunately vision may never be as sharp following surgery as it was before, even when prescription glasses are worn.

Floaters

Close one eye and look up at a blue sky. The shapes you see, the jagged specks, little lines, spider webs or circles floating in your field of vision are called floaters. Virtually every adult has them. Floaters are actually small clumps of gel that form in the vitreous of the eye, the jellylike substance that fills the chamber behind the lens of the eye. Nothing can be done to stop the progressive liquefaction of the vitreous gel inside the eye. Condensations in the gel that cast shadows on the retina, which we call "floaters," are expected in later life.

Treatment

If you've been aware of floaters in your eye for a long time, there is no cause for alarm. These "little friends" are trapped in the vitreous jelly of the eye and just drift randomly from one side to the other. Most floaters are quite benign, and there is no practical cure for them. From time to time they may bother you when you're reading, or if they happen to appear directly in your line of vision. To make them go away, just look up and down several times. This movement within the eye will cause the floaters to do just that, float, and your vision will return to normal.

Cause for Concern

Most floaters and flashes are no cause for alarm. A sudden shower of floaters, however, is more ominous and could indicate a tear in the retina with blood casting the shadows instead of the vitreal gel opacities.

Because the sudden onset of flashes and floaters may be a symptom of a retinal tear and impending detachment of the retina, the retina should be immediately checked by an ophthalmologist if this occurs.

Only rarely does the examination reveal a tear. But if it does, laser treatment or freezing (cryotherapy) can prevent the tear progressing to a retinal detachment. Once the line-of-sight retina is detached, even if it is reattached with surgery, permanent loss of sharp vision may occur.

If the retina is detaching, an area of blindness will spread, like a curtain being drawn, over the field of vision. Starting far off to the side, it will spread toward the line of sight until the eye becomes totally blind.

WHAT TO DO

- Move your eyes up and down several times. This will cause floaters to drift away from your line of vision.

- See your ophthalmologist for a complete examination if you notice a sudden shower of floaters accompanied by flashing light. This may signal a retinal tear or detachment and requires immediate treatment.

PINK EYE

Richard D. Lester, M.D.

Dr. Lester is clinical instructor of Ophthalmology,
Columbia University College of Physicians and Surgeons in New York City

"Pink eye" is a term usually used to mean either a viral or bacterial infection that affects the conjunctiva, the thin transparent lubricating tissue that lines the eyes and the inside of the eyelids. Whenever the conjunctiva becomes red and inflamed, or this redness is combined with a mucus discharge from the eye, the condition is popularly called pink eye.

Although it is not usually a serious eye ailment, pink eye is quite common and can be bothersome for both children and adults. Typical symptoms include the giveaway pink or reddish tinge to the white of the eye and a sandy or gritty sensation that you feel when you blink. Some people may also feel an itching sensation or a dryness in the eye.

If pink eye is caused by a bacterial infection, a yellow or white discharge is often found in the eye. When you wake up, the eyelashes are usually stuck together by the dried pus. There may also be a "bogginess" or heaviness felt around the eyes and some low-grade pain or soreness. If the whites of both your eyes are red, but there is little or no discharge, this is more symptomatic of a viral infection.

The eyes are so susceptible to infection because they're not sterile, and rely on lysozyme, an enzyme found in the tears, to destroy bacteria. Bacteria line the surface of the eyelids, all the way down into the shaft of the eyelashes, which makes the conjunctiva predisposed to germs.

The pink eye virus or bacteria are also commonly picked up by shaking hands with an infected person and then touching your fingers to your face. The bacteria or virus can easily travel this way to the eye. The incubation period for pink eye is hard to determine, but it could be a day or two.

Treatment

To relieve any accompanying symptoms of dryness, lubricating eye drops should be used. These are purchased over-the-counter at any pharmacy.

A warm compress speeds healing. Dip a clean washcloth in warm water, gently wring it out, and place it over the eyes for 5 minutes. When the compress cools, apply another warm one. Repeat the procedure two or three times throughout the day.

If you're still bothered by the condition on the second day, consult your physician.

When you have pink eye, certain precautions are paramount because some eye infections are highly contagious and easily spread by the hands or direct contact. Wash your hands after you've touched the eye area. Don't ever share a towel or washcloth; use your own. When you dab your eyes to clean away the discharge, use tissues and throw them away immediately afterward.

Pink eye is not to be confused with allergic conjunctivitis. This disorder is caused by specific allergies to various pollens or cosmetics. Pollen allergies typically affect both eyes, causing extreme itchiness and redness. Sneezing is also a common symptom. This condition is best treated by first identifying the specific pollen triggers and then avoiding them. Over-the-counter antihistamines provide adequate short-term relief for the itching.

If a cosmetic is the suspected culprit, test the cosmetic in one eye to see if it triggers pink eye. If it does, avoid that product.

Toxic conjunctivitis, also called environmental conjunctivitis, will also redden the whites of the eyes. This is not an eye infection but a reaction to various chemical vapors or fumes such as ammonia, chlorinated pool water, or cigarette smoke. For relief, flush the eyes with warm water and stay away from the irritants.

Cause for Concern

Your ophthalmologist should be consulted if a thick milky ooze collects on the eyelids or if the eyelashes are crusted with dried pus. This is usually an indicator of bacterial infection and prescription medication will probably be needed. If your condition continues longer than several weeks, additional prescription medication may be recommended to relieve symptoms, or you may need to consult an allergist to find the cause of a suspected allergic reaction.

What the Doctor Will Do

During an eye exam, the doctor will check your allergic history and general health, look in the eyes for discharge, and check for the inflamed conjunctiva. Many times, antibiotic eye drops will be prescribed. In five to seven days the condition should begin to clear up. If not, antibiotics may need to be stopped or changed, and the eye discharge cultured. The doctor will also check for any reaction to the medication or presence of resistant bacteria.

WHAT TO DO

- Place a warm compress repeatedly over the eyes for 5 minutes. Repeat the procedure two to three times throughout the day.
- Wash hands after you touch your face.
- Don't share towels or washcloths.
- Carefully dispose of tissues used to clean around the eyes.

STYE

Mitchell H. Friedlaender, M.D.

Dr. Friedlaender is an ophthalmologist at the
Scripps Clinic and Research Foundation, La Jolla, California

A stye is an inflammation of one of the many eyelash follicles or glands on the eyelid margin, and is typified by a red, tender, often painful bump that is usually not infectious. Sometimes the stye may appear to be swollen and whitish on top, like a pimple, but it may also be so deep in the gland that it won't come to a head at all.

Styes develop when an eyelid gland that secretes oil or tears becomes sluggish, a genetic condition that's the most common cause of the problem, or else when one of the many eyelid glands becomes clogged with oil or dirt due to poor hygiene.

Although the condition is found in people of all ages and groups, styes are especially common among those of Scottish, Irish, and English descent. These people often have fair complexions, with prominent glands in the eyelids, nose, and forehead.

Treatment

Over 90 percent of styes will go away when treated with a hot compress and a light massage of the stye with the fingers to express the pus. Heat brings the secretions to the surface and opens up the gland. Massage also encourages movement to the surface.

To prepare a hot compress, take a clean washcloth and place it in water that's as hot as you can tolerate without burning yourself. Wring out the cloth and place it on the stye for 5 minutes. Repeat three to four times daily for one to two weeks. Each time, follow the compress with a gentle massage of the stye.

If the stye is on the upper lid, gently massage downward with your index finger. Don't press too hard. For styes on the lower lid, massage upward to move the secretions to the surface. When the pus does finally discharge, carefully wash the eyelid area.

Cause for Concern

If you still have a stye after two weeks of home treatment, see your physician, who will decide if surgical draining is needed.

What the Doctor Will Do

The doctor will use a local anesthetic, lance the stye from the inside of the lid and drain out the material. In most cases an antibiotic ointment will be applied and an eye patch will be worn for twenty-four hours to avoid infection.

WHAT TO DO

- Apply a hot compress for 10 minutes three to four times daily.
- A stye can be gently massaged to express it. For styes on the upper lid, gently mas-

sage downward. Massage upward for styes on the lower lid. When the pus discharges, wash the eyelid carefully.

- If the stye doesn't clear up in two weeks, it may need to be drained. See your physician.

The Ear

GENERAL INFORMATION

The ear is a complex, three-part organ of hearing and balance. The outer or external ear is the part you can see. The outer ear canal is the ¾-inch passage that conducts sound waves to the eardrum. Too much water in the outer ear can break down the protective earwax and cause an infection of the ear canal called swimmer's ear. Anytime wax builds up here, it can lead to a "clogged" feeling or earache.

The middle ear, the small cavity between the eardrum and inner ear, houses three little bones that conduct sound from the eardrum to the inner ear. Bacterial and viral infection are by far the most common problems of the middle ear and must be

continued on page 27

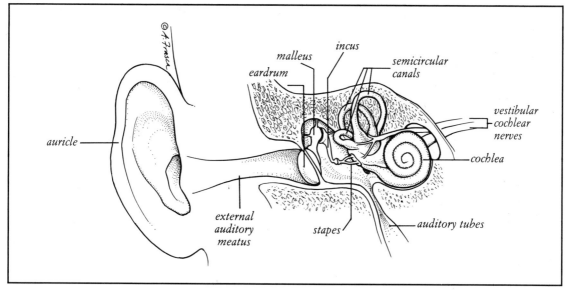

COMMON EAR PROBLEMS

AIRPLANE EARS
The temporary inability of the Eustachian tube to compensate adequately for atmospheric changes in the middle ear during aircraft descents or scuba diving (barotrauma) causes this often painful condition. Symptoms include fullness in the ear and earache.   **Page 27**

DIZZINESS (VERTIGO)
Symptoms range from mild to severe, lasting from seconds to days. Episodes of dizziness may be triggered by many causes.   **Page 34**

EARACHE
Dull, throbbing, or sharp pain in one or both ears typically signals an infection or a temporomandibular joint (TMJ) problem.   **Page 29**

EARWAX
Discomfort is brought on by oversecretion of wax, or by wax manually pushed up against the eardrum. Cotton tipped applicators are the biggest offenders. Clogged feeling and partial hearing loss are symptoms. May require medical treatment.   **Page 31**

SWIMMER'S EAR
An itchy and usually painful infection of the ear canal caused by excessive moisture, which breaks down the protective skin and earwax barrier.
                   Page 33

treated by a physician. The Eustachian tube, which helps regulate air pressure, is located in the middle ear and leads to the back of the throat and nose.

The inner ear contains the organ for hearing and balance. Any disorder here is considered serious and must be treated by a physician.

EAR SPECIALISTS

OTOLARYNGOLOGIST (M.D.). An otolaryngologist is a doctor trained to treat disorders of the ear, nose, and throat. Often called an ear, nose, and throat (ENT) specialist.

EAR EMERGENCIES

HEMORRHAGE. Bleeding in the middle ear often occurs after a blow to the head, and can be a sign of a skull fracture. Place a sterile gauze pad over the ear and transport the person to the hospital Emergency Department.

LACERATION. If the external ear has been cut or torn, place a sterile gauze pad over the ear. Wrap detached pieces of the ear in a cold, moist towel and place in a container of ice. Contact your physician and go directly to the hospital Emergency Department.

PHYSICIAN'S CARE REQUIRED

RUPTURED EARDRUM. A blow to the ear, changes in air pressure from diving (squeeze injury) or flying, improper ear cleaning, explosions, and infection of the middle ear may cause a hole in the eardrum. Symptoms include pain, hearing loss, and a slight blood discharge. Ruptures often heal by themselves, but after examination, antibiotics may be prescribed to prevent infection.

AIRPLANE EARS

Noel L. Cohen, M.D.

*Dr. Cohen is professor and chairman of Otolaryngology,
New York University School of Medicine in New York City*

Many flyers are afflicted with barotitis media, or airplane ears, the partial hearing loss, annoying earache, and "clogged up" feeling you experience during a plane's descent. Any one of these symptoms may range in intensity from mildly uncomfortable to extremely painful.

The cause of airplane ears is well understood: the eardrum retracts to changes in pressure in the airplane cabin, and the Eustachian tube cannot open properly to equalize the pressure that builds on either side of the eardrum. The Eustachian tube helps drain secretions from the middle ear into the throat, and also exchanges air between the ears and nose. When there is a pressure differential, as there is in flying or scuba diving, the Eustachian tube compensates by allowing a little more extra air to be pumped into or out of the middle ear. This is sometimes difficult to do, and it's made more difficult when you have a cold or allergy, since the lining of the tube becomes swollen.

Treatment

First, avoid drinking alcoholic beverages in-flight. Alcohol causes the mucus membranes to become engorged and the Eustachian tube to swell.

Once the "Fasten Seatbelt" signs start flashing and the plane begins its descent to the airport, swallow several times. This helps keep the Eustachian tube open and equalizes pressure in the ear.

If this doesn't work, blow your nose—again, an attempt to keep the Eustachian tube open. Yawning or chewing gum are also follow-up strategies. The goal is to have a little droplet of air pass from the nose and throat into the middle ear to relieve the pressure.

Another method to unblock the ears is to squeeze the nostrils shut with thumb and forefinger, inhale through the mouth, and then attempt to force the air back into the nose. You know your ears have unclogged when you feel them pop. Often this popping sensation is accompanied by a mild pain, but it vanishes quickly.

Never try to avoid airplane ears by sleeping through a descent because the pressure in the ears still continue, asleep or not. Sleeping only robs you of the ability to take positive steps to prevent airplane ears, and when you land, you'll find yourself in great discomfort.

Cause for Concern

The potential for danger develops when you fly with a cold or allergy, both of which can elevate ear pain. In rare instances, this can lead to a hemorrhage of the middle ear.

Try to avoid flying whenever you have a cold. The clogged feeling you typically get as the plane descends is magnified tremendously by this respiratory problem. If you must fly when you have a cold, take an over-the-counter decongestant tablet one hour before landing in order to reduce the swelling in the lining of your Eustachian tube and nasal passages. (Caution: many decongestants contain pseudoephedrine, which stimulates the central nervous system and can pose problems for heart patients. Sometimes it can also lead to mild insomnia.)

For those who suffer pain from airplane ears on a regular basis, take an OTC decongestant even in the absence of cold symptoms. Allergy sufferers, in particular, should take all their medication as prescribed. I always carry a decongestant nose spray, and if I've had a recent cold, I spray both nostrils an hour prior to landing. An OTC spray works fine.

If your infant or child has a cold or allergy, consult with your pediatrician before flying. An assessment will have to be made regarding the child's readiness to fly, and medication may have to be prescribed so the child can travel safely and comfortably. A child's still-developing Eustachian tube/middle ear complex may be unable to handle the atmospheric changes without the medicine, and the resulting ear pain can be excruciating. During descent, make sure infants and children are sitting upright to maximize the Eustachian tube opening. Also, give the baby a bottle during descent. The swallowing should help relieve pressure.

What the Doctor Will Do

If you fly frequently and often experience pain that lasts long after your flight, consult with an ear specialist. In extreme cases, the eardrum may have to be lanced to equalize the pressure. Although it is unusual to reach this point, it's far from rare.

If you fly often and the self-help measures don't work, a ventilation tube may have to be inserted into one or both of your middle ears to keep the air passage open at all times. It may be a dramatic step, but it's the only recourse. These tubes are identical to the ones used in children with chronic ear infections.

WHAT TO DO

- Avoid all alcoholic beverages in-flight.
- Swallow several times as the plane descends.
- Blow your nose.
- Chew gum or suck on candy.
- Squeeze your nostrils shut, gulp in air through your mouth. Try to force the air into your nose.
- Take over-the-counter decongestants an hour before your flight is due to land or use a nose spray. If you have allergies, take your medication before flying.
- Consult with a physician prior to flight time if your baby or young child has a cold or allergies.
- If you still have ear difficulties and travel frequently, consult with an ear specialist.

EARACHE

Michael E. Glasscock III, M.D.

Dr. Glasscock is clinical professor of Otolaryngology and assistant clinical professor of Neurosurgery at the Vanderbilt University School of Medicine in Nashville, Tennessee

Earache pain can range in severity from a mild, dull ache that doesn't seem to let up, to an intense searing pain felt in front of, above, or behind the ear.

By far, the most common cause of earache is a bacterial infection in the middle ear, brought on by a cold or flu. This requires antibiotic treatment and should be cleared up in fourteen days. Although pain relief is immediate, the full course of antibiotic therapy must be continued to eliminate the underlying infection completely.

The infection of swimmer's ear (see SWIMMER'S EAR, page 33) can also cause intense ear pain, but in most cases, when detected early, it can be treated effectively at home. However, if pain become unbearable, see your doctor.

After infection, TMJ (an abbreviation for TEMPOROMANDIBULAR JOINT SYNDROME, see page 107), is the most common cause of earache. This joint is located right in front of the ear canal and when it acts up, you feel referred pain directly in the ear. TMJ is a painful condition that usually requires medical attention.

Of course, there are some benign causes of earaches. Exposure to extreme cold will numb your ears, and they will eventually pulsate with excruciating pain. A hat that covers your ears will alleviate this problem quite handily.

Earaches can also be caused by changing air pressure in an airplane (see AIRPLANE EARS, page 27) or by scuba diving. This can often be treated with basic self-help measures described on page 28.

Treatment

Prior to seeking medical attention, do the following things to help relieve pain symptoms associated with an earache:

Take your temperature to see if you have a fever. A fever is often a sign that the body is fighting an infection. Two aspirin tablets should help ease the earache pain. Because of the risk of Reye's syndrome, however, children under twelve should be given acetaminophen, either in liquid or tablet form.

Drop baby oil, brought to body temperature, into the sore ear. Warm oil doesn't treat the cause of the earache, but it may offer some relief before you get to see a doctor.

Another remedy for the pain is a heating pad. Don't put it on the highest setting because this can harm the outer ear. Keep it on low setting to provide warmth and help diminish the ache.

If you don't have a heating pad available, use a hair dryer instead. Set it on low and hold it at least 18 inches from the head. Let the warm air go directly into the ear.

Cause for Concern

Earaches aren't common for adults, so they should be taken seriously when they do occur. Some adult ear pain can be caused by referred pain from another part of the body. For example, a malignancy in the nasal pharynx is known to cause earaches.

Babies often signal ear pain by pulling on their earlobes, tilting their heads to one side, and crying uncontrollably.

Infants and children are more prone to earaches because their still-developing Eustachian tubes can't drain excess fluids properly from the ear, and infection sets in quite easily. Children in day care, play groups, and preschool, in particular, pick up an inordinate number of infections due to high exposure to colds, flu, and viral and bacterial infection rampant in those populations. Normally, by age eight, the Eustachian tubes function well, and earache frequency diminishes dramatically, if not entirely.

Whenever young children have earaches, they should be examined by a doctor as soon as possible. In addition to infection, ear pain could be a symptom of something more ominous, such as meningitis, an inflammation of the brain and spinal column. If left unchecked, an ear infection could lead to mastoiditis, a serious inflammation of the middle ear that may eventually require corrective surgery.

In some instances, an untreated ear infection may go on to rupture the eardrum. This may actually provide pain relief, but the physician's aim is to stop the infection with antibiotics before it reaches this stage. If the eardrum does rupture, it's not necessarily a cause for alarm. In fact, in most cases it will heal itself within one to two weeks without damaging the ear or causing hearing loss. Prior to antibiotic therapy, doctors routinely made a slit in the eardrum to relieve pain caused by a buildup of pressure and fluid. The procedure is called a myringotomy.

WHAT TO DO

- Take two acetaminophen (for children under twelve) or two aspirin or ibuprofen tablets.
- Place a heating pad on your ear.
- Place a few drops of body-temperature baby oil into the ear.
- See your doctor. If earache pain is too much to bear and you can't wait to see your physician, go directly to a hospital Emergency Department for immediate treatment.

EARWAX

Yosef F. Krespi, M.D.

Dr. Krespi is the director of the Ear, Nose, Throat Service, St. Luke's/Roosevelt Hospital Center, New York City, and professor of Otolaryngology, Columbia University College of Physicians and Surgeons

Cerumen, or earwax, the yellow-orange substance found in your outer ear, can cause serious problems when it's oversecreted and builds up excessively in the ear, or when it is pushed deep into the ear canal. This often leads to discomfort and a feeling of "fullness" in the ear.

Pain of varying intensity often accompanies wax buildup and a diminution of hearing is not uncommon. In rare instances, even balance problems develop when wax bulges against the eardrum.

Earwax is normally secreted by glands in the outer portion of the ear canal. The main function of wax is to lubricate the canal, protecting the skin from infection and other conditions. Typically, the wax is secreted, then flakes off, and starts to move out of the ear. However, buildup occurs when the wax inexplicably moves inward instead.

Treatment

Many times, earwax problems are self-induced. Often, wax is packed into a ball and pushed inward with a cotton-tip applicator. To remove the wax safely, the ear should be irrigated with a special solution, or, when that fails, a doctor must take it out with a special instrument.

A good way to prevent wax problems is to clean and dry your ears methodically. I don't allow Q-Tips or any other kind of cotton-tip applicator in my household, because I find that their misuse is a major cause of problems. Cliché the expression may be, but never put anything smaller than your elbow into your ear. After every shower, I dry the outer surface of my ears with cotton balls. This is a very effective way to remove wax that has flaked off into the outer ear. It also prevents its being pushed back in.

Some people have a tendency to produce an overabundance of earwax. For them, I recommend an effective, safe, and natural homemade remedy for softening and removing excess wax.

Make a solution of $\frac{1}{3}$ hydrogen peroxide and $\frac{2}{3}$ water. Add 2 tablespoonfuls of glycerin. (Glycerin, an inexpensive by-product of soap that acts as the lubricating agent in the mixture, is available over-the-counter in any pharmacy.) Make sure the solution is at body temperature, or else it will cause dizziness as it enters the ear canal. Use the front portion of your forearm to assess temperature, as is done when feeding infants.

Shake up the ingredients and put into a good size rubber bulb syringe—20 cc or 50 cc. Holding it in front of the ear canal, and without pushing it in any farther, irrigate the ear, aiming the solution toward the upper portion of the ear canal.

Give the syringe a gentle, continuous squeeze, repeating the rinsing two or three times per session. That should loosen built-up earwax and cause it to come out. Avoid any unnecessary mess by performing the wash in a tub, shower, or over the sink.

The wash sessions may be repeated daily for two or three days. This will do several things: If the built-up wax is dry, the glycerin mixture will soften it. Even if you are unsuccessful on the first or second day, the wax may eventually loosen enough to come out.

Cause for Concern

If nothing happens after three days of ear rinsing with this solution, it's time to see an ear specialist for wax removal.

Earwax comes in many textures. For some people it may be very soft and easy to wash out, while others may have rock-hard wax, and no matter how many times it's washed, it doesn't seem to soften. This is the wax that needs to be removed by an ear doctor.

If you develop pain, swelling, tenderness over the ear cartilage, persistent hearing loss, and milky discharge, this may be a sign of ear infection. See your ENT specialist.

WHAT TO DO

- Don't use cotton-tip applicators for cleaning your ears.
- Clean and dry your outer ears with cotton balls after bathing.
- Use an ear wash when wax buildup becomes a problem.
- If earwax is a chronic problem, see your ear specialist for a checkup and treatment.

SWIMMER'S EAR

Berkeley S. Eichel, M.D.

Dr. Eichel is clinical professor of Otolaryngology, UCLA School of Medicine in Los Angeles, California

External otitis, or swimmer's ear, starts out as a nagging itch, brought on by a softening of the protective lining of the ear canal. However, it can blossom into as painful an infection as you will ever experience. For adults, swimmer's ear is the second most common cause of ear pain after TMJ syndrome (see TMJ, page 107). With a few simple preventive measures it can be kept in check, never developing into a full-blown infection.

Swimmer's ear is a problem that affects anyone who spends time in water, lives in a humid environment, or sweats profusely. Water and excessive moisture wash away the ear canal's protective skin and earwax barrier and create a medium for bacterial growth. Contrary to popular belief, swimming in dirty water does not necessarily bring on swimmer's ear. When the skin-and-wax barrier is intact, it repels bacteria.

Pool swimmers are particularly at risk because the water-chlorine combination changes ear chemistry from an acidic medium to an alkaline one. Once again, this creates a perfect breeding ground for bacteria.

Surprisingly, using cotton-tip applicators to clean the ears is the leading cause of external otitis. A few twists with an applicator is all it takes to rub away protective skin and earwax in the canal.

Although swimmer's ear may appear to come on suddenly, it usually has been building for some time. An obvious early symptom is itching, although some people may experience a secretion of clear liquid.

Treatment

The best way to combat the itch of swimmer's ear is with strict aural hygiene. This means using alcohol ear drops to treat and prevent the condition. The alcohol ear drops not only kill fungus and bacteria, but help restore the normal acid base in the ear, which in turn makes it difficult for bacteria to multiply. Look for over-the-counter ear drops such as Swim-Ear at any pharmacy. These drops contain 3 percent boric acid in isopropyl alcohol.

To make your own alcohol ear drops, mix up a solution containing 1 part white vinegar and 1 part rubbing alcohol. Warm the container with the solution to body temperature by holding it in your hands.

Tilt your head downward, with your affected ear up. Place several drops into the ear with an eyedropper and let them remain for thirty seconds. Tilt your head to the side and let the mixture drain out. Repeat three times daily. In seven days the condition should be cleared up. Continue using the drops once daily for the next month. If you are a daily swimmer, wear a swim cap and use the drops after each workout.

Cause for Concern

When swimmer's ear is unchecked and advances into an infection, extreme pain, yellowish pus, and even temporary hearing loss can occur. At this point it must be treated by a physician who will clean out the ear, and administer antibiotic ear drops or pain medication, or both. If the conditions keeps recurring, the doctor will take a culture to find the exact cause and begin a new round of treatment.

When you suspect you may be suffering from swimmer's ear and the pain in your ear becomes unbearable, before you see your doctor, take 2 acetaminophen, ibuprofen, or aspirin tablets.

Practice good aural hygiene: Leave your ears alone. Don't use cotton-tip applicators to clean or dry your ears, and don't rub them vigorously with a towel. Instead, use cotton balls or a hair dryer set on low.

Do not use ear plugs. A common misconception about ear plugs is that they keep water out of the ears. I don't think they do a good job, and I don't recommend their use. Ear plugs are actually meant to attenuate sound, and are not very effective in keeping your ears dry. Moisture that does seep into the ear canal gets trapped there, eventually creating an environment that's quite suitable for swimmer's ear. To keep your ears dry, wear a bathing cap.

WHAT TO DO

- Do not use ear plugs when you swim; wear a cap instead.
- Use alcohol ear drops regularly if you are prone to swimmer's ear; live in a warm, moist climate; or swim on a regular basis.

DIZZINESS (VERTIGO)

Ronald J. Tusa, M.D., Ph.D.

Dr. Tusa specializes in Neuro-Otology and is associate professor of Neurology and Otolaryngology/Head and Neck Surgery at the Johns Hopkins Hospital in Baltimore, Maryland

Dizziness is a broad term that's used to describe many different conditions, including vertigo. Vertigo is the sensation of the room spinning around you, or of being pushed through space for short periods as everything near you remains stationary. This perception is usually associated with nausea and vomiting.

Dizziness is one of the most common medical complaints for Americans over sixty-five, and injuries due to dizziness result in more than half of the accidental deaths of people in this age group. In many instances dizziness can be triggered by a certain medication, an ear infection, a blow to the head, a migraine disorder, or inner ear degeneration. In addition, psychological problems due to anxiety and depression also cause dizziness.

Symptoms of dizziness can range from

mild to severe, can occur frequently or very rarely, and they can last for just a brief moment or continue for days.

Some mild forms of dizziness can often be successfully treated with home remedies, medication, or a combination of the two. Others, such as balance disorder, sustained vertigo, and sustained lightheadedness require a visit to a medical specialist for proper diagnosis and treatment. Whenever you feel dizzy, sit or lie down and rest for a while.

Benign Paroxysmal Positional Vertigo

One of the most common types of vertigo is "benign paroxysmal positional vertigo (BPPV)." Benign means that there is nothing seriously wrong, while paroxysmal means the dizziness comes on suddenly. BPPV typically develops when tiny gravity-sensing granules in the inner ear move into areas where they shouldn't be.

The first tip-off to BPPV may be a brief (less than 1 minute) attack of vertigo when turning over or lying down in bed, or when moving the head to look at something on a high shelf.

Treatment

After being properly diagnosed by an otolaryngologist or neurologist with a special interest in dizziness, BPPV is easily treated in the doctor's office or with special home exercises that will cure the ailment permanently, sometimes in a matter of days, oftentimes within two weeks.

To perform the home exercises, sit on the side of a bed and lean to the right side so the right ear is down on the bed. If you are having problems with your right ear, you will quickly become dizzy, perhaps even nauseous. Wait 20 seconds until the dizziness stops and then sit straight up. Wait 20 seconds, then lean over on your left side so your left ear is on the bed. Wait 20 seconds and then sit up. Perform this exercise ten to fifteen times, three times a day.

No one is certain why this drill causes dizziness to go away, but it's thought that the brain comes to recognize that there is a motion problem and begins to compensate for it. Or it may just be a matter of finally being able to move the debris out of the semicircular canal.

Lightheadedness

Lightheadedness is a common form of dizziness that is due to the decrease of blood flow to the brain. Symptoms include a feeling of faintness or giddiness.

Temporary low blood pressure (orthostatic hypotension) is the most common cause of lightheadedness. It develops when you rapidly stand up from a lying or sitting position. Blood pools in the feet and ankles, and blood pressure drops, momentarily depriving the brain of oxygen.

Low blood pressure is frequently a morning occurrence for the elderly when they get out of bed, or on hot days when the blood vessels become dilated. It's also common for most people after taking a hot shower or bath. This form of lightheadedness can also be caused after drinking alcohol or after taking sedatives or medication for depression or high blood pressure. If it happens often, it can be a cause for concern.

Treatment

If you are prone to this problem, the best remedy after awakening is to avoid rapid or sudden change of posture. Sit at the edge of the bed for ten to twenty seconds. Hold on to the side of the bed and then slowly start to stand up. Perform this same routine when arising from a chair.

Also, check your blood pressure while lying down and again while standing. If there is more than a 20 mm Hg drop when standing, inform your physician. This difference in lying and standing blood pressure may be age-related, or related to nerve damage (neuropathy) caused by alcohol or diabetes mellitus (excessive sugar in the blood). Your doctor will review your medication and daily diet to determine the cause of lightheadedness.

If you often become lightheaded after taking a hot shower or bath, then it's best to end your bathing with cooler water to constrict the blood vessels, and then carefully get out of the tub. If you still feel lightheaded, avoid overly hot baths and showers altogether.

Motion Sickness

Motion sickness is a form of dizziness brought on when information about movement transmitted by the inner ear to the brain is not the same as the information gathered by the eyes. For example, sitting in a moving plane, boat, bus, train, or car without viewing the passing scenery triggers the movement-sensing capacity of the ears but not of the eyes. When this sensory mismatch occurs, the brain becomes confused, and nausea, dizziness, cold sweats, headaches, and vomiting may result.

Treatment

The way that I deal with motion sickness is to sit as far forward in a moving vehicle as possible and look out the window. If you find reading in a moving vehicle triggers your motion sickness, then don't read. Focus your attention forward.

If you continually feel nauseated when traveling as a passenger in a moving vehicle, and it interferes with your enjoyment of the trip, the next time you plan a long journey, take a motion sickness pill—meclizine hydrochloride or dimenhydrinate—an hour before your trip, and another one four hours later. These two antihistamine medications are available OTC.

Scopolamine, a strong prescription medication, also works well. It is the most effective for relieving the motion sickness symptoms of astronauts and ocean racing sailors. The medication is contained in a special adhesive patch worn behind the ear. Placed on the skin four hours before a trip, the drug is automatically administered in low dosages through the skin for up to three days.

Cause for Concern

If the dizzy spell is accompanied by blurred vision, muscle weakness, numbness, or hearing loss, contact your physician immediately. Also, if you have recurrent bouts of dizziness, contact your physician or go directly to a medical center that specializes in the treatment of dizziness.

To contact a specialist in your area or make an appointment at a center in your region which specializes in dizziness, contact the Vestibular Disorders Association, 1015 N.W. 22nd Avenue, Portland, Oregon 97210, Tel: 1-503-229-7705.

WHAT TO DO

Certain types of vertigo (benign paroxysmal positional vertigo, more commonly known as BPPV), lightheadedness, and motion sickness can often be successfully treated at home and without medication.

To treat symptoms of vertigo from BPPV:

- Obtain a proper diagnosis from an otolaryngologist or neurologist.
- Sit on the side of a bed and perform the special BPPV exercises three times daily.

To prevent the sensation of lightheadedness that comes from decreased blood flow to the brain:

- Avoid any rapid change of posture.
- End your bathing with cooler water in order to constrict the blood vessels.

- Avoid overly hot baths and showers altogether if you still feel lightheaded.
- Have your blood pressure checked while lying down and then while standing. Contact your physician if there is more than a 20 mm Hg drop when standing.

To avoid or reduce the incidence of motion sickness, the feelings of dizziness and nausea brought on by an imbalance in the vestibular-ocular reflex:

- Sit as far forward in a moving vehicle as possible.
- Keep eyes focused forward. Look out a window to open space.
- Don't read in a moving vehicle.
- Take a motion sickness pill before a long journey.
- If dizziness is accompanied by a headache, blurred vision, muscle numbness, nausea, or hearing loss, contact your physician immediately.

The Digestive System

GENERAL INFORMATION

The body's highly complex digestive system performs various tasks in the breakdown and absorption of foods and the elimination of wastes.

At some time, everyone will experience difficulty within this 28-foot-long gastrointestinal tract. However, most often the ailments that arise are preventable and can be self-treated with safe and effective measures.

DIGESTIVE SPECIALISTS

GASTROENTEROLOGIST (M.D.). A gastroenterologist is an internist who specializes in the diagnosis and medical treatment of gastrointestinal disorders.

COLORECTAL SURGEON (M.D.). This medical doctor specializes in the treatment of colon and rectal disorders and performs surgery.

DIGESTIVE SYSTEM EMERGENCIES

APPENDICITIS. Inflammation and swelling of the appendix, the small pouch attached to the large intestine, which leads to severe abdominal pain in the lower right side. Vomiting, constipation, and fever are common. Do not take a laxative; appendix may rupture. Go directly to the hospital Emergency Department or contact your physician. Surgery required.

PERITONITIS. Inflammation of the abdominal cavity lining caused by bacterial infection or underlying, untreated disease such as an ulcer or appendicitis. Severe abdominal pain, fever, nausea, and vomiting are symptoms. Emergency surgery may be necessary.

COMMON DIGESTIVE PROBLEMS

BELCHING
A normal response of venting excessive gas, typically caused by taking too much air into the stomach while eating, drinking, or swallowing.   **Page 42**

CONSTIPATION
When insufficient fiber is eaten or physical activity limited, a change in bowel habits results, producing hard, small, often painful stools.   **Page 43**

DIARRHEA
Excess gas, stomach cramps, and frequent bowel movement, typically of soft or liquid feces. Diarrhea is most often triggered by bacterial or viral infections, tension, medication, or several different illnesses. Poses health danger because of dehydration.   **Page 46**

FLATULENCE
Intestinal gas caused by the breakdown of certain foods in the intestines, carbonated beverages, or excessive air swallowing.   **Page 49**

FOOD POISONING
A mild-to-severe, often transitory condition that results from consuming foods or liquids contaminated by various bacteria, viruses, or molds. May require medical attention or hospitalization.   **Page 51**

HEARTBURN
Gastroesophageal reflux is typified by occasional burning in the stomach and esophagus due to overeating; eating greasy, fat-laden foods; alcohol; tobacco; or chocolate.   **Page 54**

HEMORRHOIDS
Swollen blood vessels in the rectum and anus, accompanied by pain, itchiness, swelling, and discomfort, sometimes bleeding.   **Page 57**

continued

HICCUPS
This usually temporary disorder has no known purpose and its cause is not fully understood. In some cases, hiccups may signal underlying lung or stomach disorders. **Page 60**

NAUSEA AND VOMITING
An often transitory condition, usually virus-triggered, that results in stomach queasiness and vomiting. May also be caused by overeating, medications, food poisoning, heart attack, or vertigo. **Page 61**

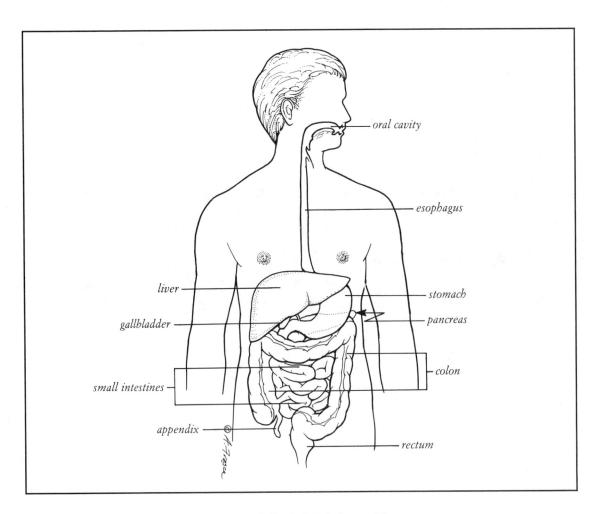

oral cavity

esophagus

liver

stomach

gallbladder

pancreas

colon

small intestines

appendix

rectum

PHYSICIAN'S CARE REQUIRED

BLOODY VOMIT, RECTAL BLEEDING, BLOOD IN THE URINE. Blood in vomit may signal a bleeding stomach ulcer. If you have not had a recent bloody nose, contact your physician. If, in addition to bloody vomit, you are sweating, your skin is cold, and you feel weak, go to the hospital Emergency Department immediately.

Rectal bleeding may be caused by hemorrhoids or gastrointestinal inflammation. Blood in the urine may signal infection or kidney problems.

CIRRHOSIS OF THE LIVER. A slow, chronic disease in which liver cells are progressively destroyed. Alcohol abuse is the most common cause. Initial symptoms are mild, but progress to weight loss, nausea, vomiting, jaundice, abdominal distention, and fatigue. The condition cannot be reversed, but medical treatment may prevent or reduce further liver damage.

GALLSTONES. A hard mass of cholesterol, bile, and calcium salts of varying shapes and sizes that collects in the gallbladder. No symptoms usually, but may cause intense pain when a stone blocks the bile duct. Pain may last for hours and is felt on the right side of the abdomen, oftentimes radiating up the back. Nausea, vomiting, and loss of appetite are also characteristic. Medication, stone fragmentation with ultrasonic sound waves, or gallbladder removal may be recommended.

GASTRITIS. Inflammation of the mucus membrane of the stomach caused by certain medications, acidic foods, excessive alcohol and food consumption, smoking, or a virus. Symptoms include nausea, diarrhea, abdominal cramps. Medications may be prescribed to reduce the amount of stomach acid.

HEPATITIS. Liver inflammation due to viral infection, excessive alcohol use, or reaction to medication such as acetaminophen, tranquilizers, or oral contraceptives. Fever, nausea, yellow discoloration of the skin (jaundice) are common symptoms. Blood test confirms diagnosis. No specific treatment, but rest and abstinence from alcohol help with recovery.

HERNIA. Protrusion of soft tissue through a tear in a weak abdominal wall muscle that causes a bulge to form. Characterized by a tender lump and discomfort. Surgery is most effective treatment.

INFLAMMATORY BOWEL DISEASE. General term for ulcerative colitis and Crohn's disease (ileitis), two chronic conditions of the intestinal tract. Cause is unknown. Symptoms include diarrhea (with blood and pus this is a sign of ulcerative colitis), fever, fatigue, weight loss, and skin lesions. Long-term medication, regulated diet, and surgery may be required.

ACUTE PANCREATITIS. Inflammation of the pancreas typified by severe pain in the mid to upper abdomen, back and chest; nausea; and vomiting that begins twelve to twenty-four hours after a large meal or excessive drinking. May also be triggered by gallstones. Medications, including antibiotics, may be administered. Hospitalization may be recommended.

ULCER. A break or hole in the lining of the stomach. Cause unknown, but smoking and alcohol play a role. Burning pain, discomfort felt in upper abdomen and lower chest may last for hours. Bleeding from stomach ulcer is rare, but may show up in stools or vomit. Prescription medications may be recommended to relieve stomach acid and help with healing.

BELCHING

Arnon Lambroza, M.D.

Dr. Lambroza is assistant professor of medicine, Cornell University Medical College, and director of the Center for Esophageal and Swallowing Disorders at the New York Hospital–Cornell Medical Center in New York City

Everyone belches or burps at one time or another to relieve excess gas buildup in the stomach. It may often be embarrassing, but for the vast majority of people, occasional belching is not a problem that needs medical attention.

Belching is triggered in two major ways. First, too much gas is produced in the stomach by eating such foods as bran, raw fruit, and vegetables, or by drinking gaseous liquids such as beer, soda, or seltzer. Even apple, grape, and prune juice can lead to belching.

The second cause is swallowing too much air, a condition known as aerophagia in chronic cases. Strange as it may seem, it doesn't take much effort to do this. Gulping your food, drinking too fast, or talking when eating brings in excessive amounts of air, which can build up in the gastrointestinal tract.

Chewing gum, sucking on candy, smoking a pipe or cigarettes, or chewing on a cigar also greatly increase air intake and, with it, belching.

Treatment

In some cases, belching is directly related to a lactose intolerance, which is the inability to break down certain sugars found in milk and milk products. A common complaint from people who are diagnosed with lactose intolerance is a feeling of being bloated and gassy.

If belching regularly occurs after drinking milk or eating a milk-based product, a simple lactose tolerance test given by a physician will quickly confirm if you are missing lactase, an essential enzyme needed to break down the sugars in milk.

Cause for Concern

There exists a chronic belching syndrome which is caused by excessive swallowing. This problem generally affects younger to middle-age women at risk for anxiety disorders. They repeatedly swallow and then, when gas and resulting pain start to build up in the stomach, they inhale more air and force themselves to burp to relieve their discomfort.

People with a chronic belching problem think they're helping themselves when they belch, but forced belching brings more air to the stomach than is expelled by belching. This swallowing-belching pattern is a vicious cycle that's extremely difficult to break.

A chronic belcher needs to address the underlying emotional turmoil that causes them to swallow so much, and seek professional help to deal constructively with it.

What the Doctor Will Do

The doctor will review the diet to check for gassy foods and drink, and point out habits such as gum chewing, smoking, and sucking on candy that can easily exacerbate belching.

In most cases, arresting the excessive swallowing will end belching.

WHAT TO DO

- Be aware of the typical foods and liquids that cause gas to build in the gastrointestinal tract.
- Take small bites when eating.
- Chew food well with the mouth closed.
- Don't talk with food in your mouth.
- Eat four to six mini-meals during the day in order to stave off feelings of extreme hunger and curb rapid eating.
- Use a glass when you drink, don't gulp or use a straw.
- Don't chew gum.
- Have a lactose tolerance test if belching regularly develops after drinking milk or eating milk products.
- If these measures fail to reduce the frequency of belching, or if you have a chronic problem, contact a gastroenterologist.

CONSTIPATION

Ira J. Schmelkin, M.D.

Dr. Schmelkin is a gastroenterologist and assistant attending physician at North Shore University Hospital in Manhasset, New York

Constipation is a common problem that is typically caused by life-style and diet. It's also a medical term whose definition varies from person to person. In essence, constipation is a decrease in *your* usual bowel movements.

Most constipation can be alleviated or prevented with simple dietary changes and regular exercise. Chronic use of laxatives plays no role in healthy bowel habits and should be eliminated.

Regular bowel patterns vary from person to person. "Normal" could be considered moving the bowels once every two to three days to as much as three times daily. Constipation occurs when your bowel movement pattern changes and fecal matter becomes hard or has reduced its mass and changed shape. It is mainly the result of nutritional deficiencies, behavioral or emotional changes, or a reduction or lack of physical activity. Much of the time, constipation is linked directly to a lack of adequate amounts of fiber in the diet.

Treatment

Fiber is roughage, the indigestible parts of whole grains, legumes, vegetables, and fruits. Once it arrives in the colon, it absorbs water, which creates soft and bulky stools, and they in turn stimulate a smoother passage to the rectum.

Unfortunately, the average American diet is woefully lacking in fiber. Americans typically consume barely 12 grams daily, well short of the 15 to 35 grams that is recommended. Meals consisting of highly processed foods and white bread that have been stripped of fiber are major reasons for this deficiency.

To eliminate and prevent constipation, gradually add more fruits, vegetables, legumes, and unprocessed whole grains to your daily diet. Also read food labels carefully to determine how much fiber they contain.

Increasing daily fiber consumption has to be gradual, however. Sudden, excessive fiber intake is not recommended because this can lead to excessive gas and bloating. Also drink plenty of water, at least 8 cupfuls daily, to provide the moisture needed to soften the stools.

If you start to feel bloated or gassy, cut back on certain beans or legumes, or else eliminate them and switch to other forms of fiber. The fiber-rich diet should start making a difference in just a day or two.

Certain medicines can bring on constipation. These include codeine-based cough preparations, calcium supplements for osteoporosis, beta-blockers, and various tranquilizers. Check with your physician if constipation develops after using any of these medicines.

Constipation may also occur when you ignore the urge to defecate. This often happens when you travel or go through emotional stress. If this retention becomes a regular practice, problems may develop with bowel control. In young elementary school children especially, constipation and accidental bowel movements may start occurring, while older people may find it increasingly more difficult to move their bowels.

If you have the urge to go to the bathroom, then go and sit on the toilet. If you have not been able to go to the bathroom for some time, then pick some quiet moment when you know you won't be rushed, and set aside 10 minutes to sit on the toilet. Read. Relax. Don't think about the bowel movement. It will occur naturally. To retrain your colon, stay for the entire 10 minutes even if you don't move your bowels.

Regular daily exercise plays a vital role in promoting good bowel functions by strengthening the muscles of the lower abdomen and pelvic floor. You don't need to become a long-distance runner or join a health club to achieve beneficial results. Walk as little as 20 minutes a day, and you will condition the muscles and help speed up the passage of food through the digestive tract. Although the average adult takes twenty-four hours to pass an entire meal through the intestines, some elite athletes take as little as one fourth the time for the same meal.

If you are bedridden for any length of time, it's not uncommon to become constipated because you lack physical movement. In that case, the use of a laxative may be in order to assist in moving the bowels.

Various laxatives are available OTC in the pharmacy. *Saline* laxatives such as milk of magnesia or citrate of magnesia work by drawing volumes of liquid into the intestine and promoting conditions similar to diarrhea. *Irritant* laxatives contain a chemical such as phenolphthalein or cascara sagrada and senna, two herbs that stimulate the intestines to secrete liquid and trigger defecation. *Mineral oil* laxatives work by coating the stool, thereby making it easier and less painful to pass out of the rectum.

Laxative use is a double-edged sword for many people. Although infrequent use will immediately help overcome constipation, frequent or chronic reliance on laxatives can upset normal peristalsis and lead to a condition known as irritable bowel syndrome.

The caffeine in regular coffee is a strong laxative that affects the nerves that stimulate intestinal contraction; thus a strong cup of coffee will quickly encourage a bowel movement in someone who doesn't drink it regularly. But the purgative effects of coffee are often diminished when it is consumed on a daily basis.

Cause for Concern

If you find that a commercial laxative doesn't help relieve constipation, or if constipation gets worse and is accompanied by abdominal pain, or if there is blood in your stool, contact your doctor.

What the Doctor Will Do

After taking a complete dietary and medical history and ruling out any complications, the doctor will make dietary suggestions. In cases of severe constipation, a laxative may be prescribed for immediate relief.

If further testing is needed, a gastroenterologist will give a barium enema and take X rays. He may also insert a flexible instrument called a sigmoidoscope into the anus to check for cancer or obstructing lesions in the colon.

WHAT TO DO

- Gradually increase daily fiber intake to 15–35 grams.
- Drink 8 glasses of water daily.
- Don't ignore or postpone the urge to defecate.
- Develop regular bowel habits.
- Exercise daily. Walking as little as 20 minutes is of great benefit.
- If constipation gets worse, even after using a laxative, or if it is accompanied by abdominal pain, or if there is blood in your stool, contact your doctor.

DIARRHEA

Ray E. Clouse, M.D.

Dr. Clouse is associate professor of medicine at the Washington University School of Medicine and director of the Digestive Disease Clinical Center of Barnes Hospital in St. Louis, Missouri

Diarrhea may occur by itself or be accompanied by excess gas, stomach cramping, nausea, vomiting, and fever. It is a symptom of underlying conditions typically caused by a virus, bacteria, parasite, or an intolerance to foods, particularly milk products. In most cases diarrhea clears up on its own within two to seven days, or once the source of the problem has been diagnosed and treated.

Some medications trigger diarrhea. These include antibiotics, high blood pressure and cholesterol-lowering drugs, digitalis, asthma medications, antacids containing magnesium, and, of course, laxatives. Consult with your physician if you suspect your medication. Contaminated foods and drink are also a major cause of diarrhea (see FOOD POISONING, page 51).

Normal bowel habits range widely: from three movements a day to three per week. Some people have chronic diarrhea and perceive it as a normal bowel movement. However, chronic diarrhea can lead to nutritional deficiencies, and should be checked out by the family physician. A change in diet or a prescription medication may eliminate the problem completely.

Treatment

Whenever I have nonspecific diarrhea stemming from a bacteria or viral flu, I drink plenty of *clear* fluids containing sugar and salt. The accent is on clear liquids to avoid substances that exacerbate diarrhea and worsen dehydration. Milk and milk products should be avoided because they often worsen diarrhea even in people whose digestive systems can normally handle dairy products. Many times the special lactase enzyme necessary for the digestion of lactose, the natural sugar found in dairy products, is temporarily destroyed by the invading virus or bacteria.

For diarrhea, drink water, caffeine-free soda such as ginger ale, fruit juice, consommé, and decaffeinated tea. For more acute diarrhea typified by five or more bowel movements a day, drink commercially prepared "sports" drinks, such as Gatorade.

To prepare your own replacement drink, mix ½ teaspoon of salt, ½ teaspoon of baking soda, and 4 tablespoons of sugar into 1 quart of water. Shake well and drink frequent, small amounts of the mixture.

For another effective rehydration drink, add ½ teaspoon of honey and a pinch of table salt to 1 cup of orange juice. In another cup filled with water, add ¼ teaspoon of baking soda. Drink the contents of the first cup, followed immediately by the contents of the second.

For infants and young children with mild or severe diarrhea, several brands of premixed rehydration solutions are available OTC. These solutions contain all the necessary electrolytes, and the child should be encouraged to drink a cup of the liquid every hour.

As you start to improve—if you don't feel nauseated—begin to eat bread or salted crackers. Then eat pasta or rice, and add chicken, fish, or beef to your diet. Fats are harder for the body to assimilate and should only be reintroduced when diarrhea has completely stopped.

If you have mild, nonbloody diarrhea and are not sick with a fever, take generic loperamide according to bottle directions. This formerly prescription-only, liquid antidiarrheal medication is available OTC in the pharmacy. It can be as effective for some people as prescription-only loperamide capsules. It is also the active ingredient in such OTC medications as Imodium A-D.

In addition to loperamide, the old diarrhea standby, bismuth subsalicylate (the active ingredient found in Pepto-Bismol), is also helpful, particularly for diarrhea caused by bacterial infection. If you are aspirin-sensitive, or already taking aspirin, consult your physician before using it because it may produce side effects.

Attapulgite (the active ingredient found in Kaopectate) has not been scientifically proven to work consistently, although some people swear by it when they have diarrhea. Loperamide is a better choice for most people.

Cause for Concern

If stools are loose and watery for more than forty-eight hours without signs of improvement, or if the diarrhea is accompanied by a fever above 101 degrees F, or if it is accompanied by severe and unremitting abdominal cramping, or if blood or mucus appears in the stools, or if diarrhea develops suddenly after taking antibiotic medication, high blood pressure or heart medication, contact your physician.

Also, if you have chronic diarrhea that lasts for several weeks accompanied by no other symptoms, seek a medical evaluation.

The doctor should also be contacted if dehydration develops because of diarrhea or associated vomiting. Dehydration is the excessive loss of body fluids and salts needed for normal metabolism through bowel movements, vomiting, or both. This can be a life-threatening condition for infants and the elderly, and can develop in a few hours.

Contact a physician immediately or head to the nearest hospital Emergency Department if you notice the following signs of dehydration: low urine production, sunken eyes and abdomen, dry "cotton" mouth, excessive thirst, lightheadedness, pale and dry skin that fails to spring back to place when gently pulled, sleepiness, or extreme lethargy.

Traveler's Diarrhea

There are well-documented areas in Africa, Asia, Latin America, and the Middle East where traveler's diarrhea is a problem for upward of 30 to 60 percent of the tourists who visit. Contrary to popular belief, it appears that eating contaminated food is the major cause of traveler's diarrhea and *not* drinking from the local water supply. Impure water can bring on diarrhea, of course, but not to the extent that was once thought.

In order to remain a healthy traveler, don't buy food from street vendors. When it comes to snacks and mealtime, if you can't cook it, boil it, or peel it, then don't eat it.

Also, in areas of high risk, be wary of the water. Don't brush your teeth with water or eat any food that has been washed in the water. Don't drink water unless it's been purified or it's bottled, and don't use any ice in your drink.

To purify your own water supply, boil the water for 3 minutes.

To prevent the spread of diarrhea and eliminate chances of reinfection, after using the bathroom, always wash your hands with soap and water.

If these preventive measures fail, and you develop diarrhea, mix up a rehydration drink (see recipes under Treatment, above) to help maintain your hydration levels.

To help reduce the frequency of the bowel movements, assuming the signs and symptoms of more severe diarrhea are not present (such as fever or bloody stool), take loperamide according to directions. Again, bismuth subsalicylate (Pepto-Bismol) can be effective; however, you need to take 2 tablespoons of the liquid eight times a day. Admittedly, 8 ounces is a lot to take in one day, but it will reduce the number of loose stools for most people.

Cause for Concern

If you have a fever above 101 degrees, bloody stools, or the number of bowel movements has not decreased in two days, contact a physician. Antibiotics may have to be prescribed. The medication will work very quickly. Although the course of the illness may not be shortened, the number of bowel movements will be reduced sharply and promptly in many cases.

WHAT TO DO

- Drink plenty of *clear* fluids containing sugar and salt.
- Stay on a liquids-only diet whenever you have frequent watery bowel movements.
- Eat pasta or rice, and then add chicken, fish, or beef to your diet once you start to feel better. Fats should be reintroduced when diarrhea has completely stopped.
- Take an OTC medication such as loperamide or bismuth subsalicyclate to retard the number of bowel movements.

In cases of diarrhea, contact your physician if you have concerns about it, or if the stools are loose and watery for more than forty-eight hours, or if diarrhea is accompanied by fever above 101 degrees F, or if there is blood or mucus in the stools, or if diarrhea is accompanied by persistent abdominal cramping.

FLATULENCE

Steven Field, M.D.

*Dr. Field is clinical assistant professor of medicine (Gastroenterology),
New York University School of Medicine in New York City*

Expelled intestinal gas, or flatulence, is one of the oldest human complaints. Although it may be embarrassing, it is usually a normal by-product of human existence. If it becomes excessive, it can usually be reduced with basic changes in the daily diet.

When you eat food, bacteria in the intestines breaks it down and causes the sugars to ferment, producing gas. You also take in considerable quantities of air when you eat and drink. This can add to the gas buildup.

Cruciferous vegetables such as cabbage, broccoli, beans, brussels sprouts, and cauliflower contain a carbohydrate called stachyose that is metabolized in the intestine to form carbon dioxide. Other foods that contribute to intestinal gas include apples, bananas, carbonated beverages, corn, cucumbers, onions, and turnips.

With the increased intake of fiber in the American diet, gas has become an unwelcome problem for many people.

Common foods rich in fiber include apricots, bran, dates, figs, lentils, peaches, pears, pineapple, pistachio nuts, popcorn, prunes, strawberries, walnuts, and whole-grain wheat, rye, and oats.

Treatment

With all dietary fiber, start low and go slow. Begin with moderate amounts of fiber in the daily diet and gradually increase their quantity over a period of time. If, after this reintroduction to the diet, these fiber-rich foods continue to disturb your system, they should be eliminated entirely.

Lactose intolerance is another cause of gas. Up to 90 percent of African Americans, Native Americans, Asians, and Mediterranean peoples (Jews, Italians, and Greeks) have low levels of intestinal lactase, an enzyme necessary for the digestion of lactose, the natural sugar found in milk.

To reduce or eliminate gas caused by lactose intolerance, go on a milk-free diet for ten days. Gradually reintroduce milk products over the next few days until you reach a comfort level. Don't exceed that level.

If eliminating dairy products is impractical, consider the commercially available lactase preparations like LactAid, which come in drop, tablet, or pretreated milk.

In many cases, swallowing excessively (see BELCHING, page 42) causes gas buildup. Anyone who chews gum or tobacco; drinks excessive amounts of soda, seltzer, or beer; gulps food when he or she eats; smokes; or talks excessively while eating is a prime candidate. People with asthma are also more likely to swallow air because of reduced lung capacity and rapid, shallow breathing.

Diet candies containing the artificial sweetener sorbitol also can cause or contribute to gas and diarrhea.

If flatulence is caused by excessive

swallowing of air, stop chewing gum, slow down when you eat, or reduce or eliminate smoking. If the swallowing is a nervous habit caused by stress or underlying emotional tension, consult your physician for counseling.

There are also OTC products that may help. I say "may" because research studies have shown that these products don't do any better than placebos in providing relief from gas. However, I have many patients who claim that these products do work. The following OTC remedies may help you ward off intestinal gas:

- Activated charcoal tablets. The charcoal will turn your stools black, but it absorbs excessive gas in the colon and may provide some relief. If you are taking any medication, consult your doctor before using charcoal. Charcoal may interfere with the absorption of medication.
- Simethicone is a chemical that helps prevent gas from forming in the stomach and intestines. Simethicone is available as a prescription item but is also found in many popular antacid preparations such as Mylicon, Maalox Plus, Mylanta II, and Gas-X. Follow label directions for proper dosage.

Cause for Concern

Contact a doctor if you notice any changes. For example, if you have been feeling fine and suddenly develop intestinal gas accompanied by abdominal distention or diarrhea that lasts for a few days, several things could be going on. An intestinal parasite you picked up in your travels could be the troublemaker. In some cases, your difficulties could be caused by irritable bowel syndrome, also known as spastic colon, a common condition that typically appears in early adulthood and is characterized by intermittent gas, diarrhea, abdominal distention, and pain. Persistent and severe flatulence or chronic abdominal discomfort and diarrhea may also be symptomatic of gallbladder problems, inflammation of the intestines such as colitis and ileitis, and cancers that affect the colon and intestinal tract.

What the Doctor Will Do

If the home remedies for intestinal gas fail to bring improvement, contact your physician. The doctor will take a history, perform a careful medical exam, and possibly one or two laboratory tests. The doctor may also recommend further diagnostic tests.

WHAT TO DO

- Avoid or greatly reduce your consumption of cruciferous vegetables such as cabbage, broccoli, beans, and cauliflower.
- Eat moderate amounts of fiber-rich foods and gradually increase their quantity over a period of time.
- If dairy products are a source of gas, restrict milk and dairy products for ten days to see if symptoms improve.
- Take activated charcoal tablets according to directions.
- Use an antacid preparation containing simethicone.

  To reduce flatulence caused by excessive swallowing of air:

- Stop chewing gum.
- Slow down when you eat.
- Reduce or eliminate smoking.

- Consult your physician if excessive swallowing is caused by stress or underlying nervous tension.
- Contact your doctor if these remedies don't work or if you suddenly develop intestinal gas accompanied by abdominal distention or diarrhea that lasts for several days.

FOOD POISONING

Diane M. Sixsmith, M.D.

Dr. Sixsmith is director of Emergency Services at New York Downtown Hospital and instructor of medicine, New York University School of Medicine in New York City

At least one of five Americans suffer food poisoning each year, and over 9,000 deaths are reported as a result. Food poisoning stems not from food additives, chemical fertilizers, or pesticides applied to food by growers or processors, but from poor food storage practices in home or restaurant kitchens that cause food to become contaminated.

The symptoms of food poisoning are many, depending on the bacterium, mold, or virus present in the food, and become evident from two hours to five days after eating tainted foods. The most common symptoms of food poisoning include diarrhea, watery stools, abdominal cramps, nausea, protracted vomiting, and fever. Most food poisoning symptoms are mild, however, and can safely be treated at home.

Treatment

To make yourself more comfortable and safely speed your recovery from food poisoning, there are many things you can do, beginning with simply getting in bed and keeping warm. By resting you remove most physical demands on your debilitated system.

Diarrhea is often the major complaint in many cases of food poisoning, and this results in a tremendous loss of body fluids and nutrients from your system. If you are not too nauseated and your stomach can hold down liquids, try to drink at least 6–8 ounces of room temperature *clear* liquid per hour. Clear liquids place a minimal demand on your overtaxed gastrointestinal system, and can include water, tea with sugar, bouillon, defizzed soda, or any of the commercially prepared fluid replacement drinks (like Gatorade) available in the supermarket.

School-age children with suspected food poisoning should drink at least 5 ounces of clear liquid every hour, and infants should drink at least an ounce of liquid every hour. Avoid apple juice because it can aggravate the situation.

Don't drink milk for several days even after diarrhea has subsided. The stomach lining hasn't been replenished with the enzymes needed to handle the lactose contained in milk and milk-based products.

There is some debate in the medical community concerning diarrhea. Some physicians say it should be allowed to continue to rid the body naturally of all contaminated material in the gastrointestinal tract, and that constant fluid intake should be maintained to prevent dehydration from occurring.

Other physicians feel that the bacteria from contaminated food is sufficiently inactivated by normal body immune mechanisms and that real disability actually comes from fluid loss brought on by diarrhea. I'm from this school of thought, so for moderate to severe diarrhea, I recommend the antidiarrheal medication called loperamide, because I find that dehydration from the diarrhea, coupled with dizziness and the frequent trips to the bathroom, can be extremely debilitating.

Loperamide is a former prescription-only, narcoticlike medication that decreases the number of stools in the bowel. It is now available in OTC compounds such as Imodium A–D. Take this liquid medication (stronger capsule formulation available by prescription only) according to directions, and diarrhea will be slowed.

Once symptoms diminish, gradually introduce soft and easily digested foods such as bananas, rice and rice cereal, applesauce, toast, and pureed chicken. When diarrhea stops and the appetite becomes stronger, slowly return to the normal diet.

Prevention

- Make every effort to keep down the growth of all bacteria in food. Keep all food clean, make sure hot food stays hot and cold food is adequately refrigerated.
- Be wary of prepared foods available at salad bars, delis, and cafeteria-style buffets.
- When you picnic, bring along bags of ice or use a cooler and vacuum bottle to keep meats, salads, milk, and milk products cold. Keep the cooler in the shade and open it as infrequently as possible.
- At home, keep the refrigerator set between 34 and 40 degrees.
- Eat all foods within two hours after cooking, within one hour if room temperature is 90 degrees or higher.
- Put all leftovers back in the refrigerator as soon as possible.
- Freeze all meats, fish, and poultry that won't be consumed within two days.
- Thaw all meats and poultry in the refrigerator and not out on a countertop. The cool refrigerator keeps bacteria from growing on the defrosting meat surface.
- Keep all animals away from foods, especially during preparation.
- Wash your hands with hot water and soap before handling foods. If you have a cut on your hand or fingers, wear gloves to eliminate any chance of food contamination.
- Use one cutting board for fruits and vegetables and a different one for meats. After cutting or preparing raw meat or poultry, wash your hands with hot water and soap.
- Wash all equipment, utensils, cutting board, and countertops after each stage of preparation, and then wash carefully again when preparation is completed.
- Cook or barbecue all chicken and pork until there is no sign of pink in the meat.
- When cooking with a microwave, be sure to rotate foods during the cooking process to ensure all parts are sufficiently

cooked. Bacteria can easily survive when cooking is uneven.

- Do not buy any eggs that are broken or cracked. Use all fresh eggs within five to seven days.
- Contaminated foods often look, smell, and taste fine. However, if food—leftovers especially—doesn't smell or look right, don't eat it.

What the Doctor Will Do

If you are usually healthy and suspect food poisoning, a call to your doctor is in order. Explain the circumstances and symptoms you're experiencing. After ruling out botulism, abdominal obstruction, side effects from medication or pregnancy, or pain from kidney stones, the doctor will reassure you that this is a mild form of food poisoning and will pass with bed rest, fluids, and a bland diet.

Cause for Concern

If your condition worsens and you become extremely dehydrated, or blood appears in your diarrhea, accompanied by unrelenting abdominal pain, then you need medical attention. Contact your doctor or head to the hospital Emergency Department.

Even with mild food poisoning, some people are at risk. These include the elderly, the very young, pregnant women, alcoholics, people taking medications to reduce stomach acid, and people with diabetes, as well as those who have immunodepressed systems. When food poisoning is suspected, the doctor should be contacted immediately.

Also, if symptoms include severe diarrhea or vomiting, with an abnormally dry tongue and pale skin, contact your doctor immediately or go to the hospital Emergency Department. Hospitalization may be required in these severe cases of dehydration.

Botulism, caused by the bacterium *Clostridium botulinum,* is a rare but potentially fatal food poisoning usually caused by eating improperly prepared home-canned vegetables, poultry, and meat. The nervous system is quickly affected, with progressively worsening symptoms, including blurred or double vision, nausea, vomiting, and difficulty in swallowing, possibly ending in paralysis and respiratory failure.

Botulism is a medical emergency, and hospitalization is required so an antitoxin can be administered.

WHAT TO DO

- Get plenty of rest.
- When nausea and vomiting have stopped, drink 6–8 ounces of clear liquids every hour. Children should drink 5 ounces and infants 1 ounce of clear liquid per hour.
- Take loperamide for moderate to severe diarrhea.
- Once symptoms have diminished, gradually begin to eat easy-to-digest foods.
- Observe proper food handling and safety precautions.
- If the afflicted person is elderly, very young, pregnant, alcoholic, has diabetes, takes stomach-acid medications, or has an immunodepressed system, contact your doctor immediately.
- Also, if you are usually healthy and suspect food poisoning but have any doubts, contact your doctor.

If your condition worsens, or you become extremely dehydrated, or blood appears in your diarrhea accompanied by unrelenting abdominal pain, contact your doctor or go to the hospital Emergency Department.

HEARTBURN

Richard A. Wright, M.D.

Dr. Wright is professor of medicine at the
University of Louisville School of Medicine in Louisville, Kentucky

Heartburn, or gastroesophageal reflux, is a common condition that affects approximately 73 million Americans annually. It typically begins with a burning sensation that starts in the upper abdomen and moves up into the chest, often making its way to the back of the throat.

Heartburn gets its name from chest pains caused by stomach acid that washes up into the esophagus. This chest pain can be confused with angina, but the heart has nothing to do with it.

Distress from heartburn is common after a meal of fat-laden or acidic foods, after taking aspirin, drinking alcohol, smoking, or eating chocolate. Obesity, pregnancy, emotional turmoil, and tension can also trigger heartburn. In general, there is no cause for concern with infrequent heartburn.

Treatment

If you have heartburn symptoms, don't try to tough it out. The discomfort of occasional heartburn can be relieved by taking an OTC antacid. These medications come in tablet, liquid, or foam, and in regular and extra-strength formulations. The active agents in antacid compounds usually consist of one or more of the following ingredients: magnesium, aluminum hydroxide, sodium bicarbonate, or the centuries-old standby, calcium carbonate.

Antacids should bring relief almost instantaneously. A recommended dose one to three hours after eating should provide varying degrees of relief. If a single dose doesn't work, the problem could be more severe, and a doctor should be called.

What actually determines the overall effectiveness of an antacid depends on what and how much you ate or imbibed, and the overall state of your gastrointestinal tract. These active chemicals buffer the accumulated acid in the stomach. This helps reduce or eliminate the burn that's felt in the esophagus. Antacids do not reduce any further acid buildup or eradicate feelings of discomfort or fullness in your stomach.

In addition, if you have high blood pressure or are on a sodium-restricted diet, don't take antacids containing sodium bicarbonate because of its high sodium content. If you have kidney problems, avoid antacids with magnesium or aluminum. Also, if you're bothered by kidney stones, don't take calcium carbonate antacids because the calcium can accelerate the problem. Calcium carbonate antacids will initially quell acid buildup, but because they contain calcium, this antacid will soon cause an increase in stomach acid.

Finally, contrary to popular belief, milk is not a recommended antidote to heartburn. A glass of milk does provide immediate relief as it goes down, but milk contains calcium and protein, and these eventually stimulate even more acid production in the stomach. This can cause a more severe heartburn to return in as little as a half hour.

A WORD OF CAUTION: In some cases, antacids and certain drugs don't mix. Tetracycline, indomethacin, and buffered and nonbuffered aspirin, iron supplements, digoxin, quinidine, Valium, and corticosteroids can adversely mix with antacids in the stomach, causing problems that are far more serious than heartburn. If you are taking any of these medications, contact your doctor before dosing yourself for heartburn.

Prevention

- If certain foods or drinks regularly bring on discomfort, avoid them. These may include oranges and grapefruit, Bloody Mary mix, onions, tomatoes and tomato-based sauces, and greasy, fat-laden, or fried meat or sauce. Red wine, after-dinner liqueurs, and peppermints are also prime causes of heartburn.
- Don't smoke. Smoking allows stomach acids to enter the esophagus. Secondary smoke may have the same effect, so eat in nonsmoking sections in restaurants whenever possible.
- Avoid caffeine. It can increase production of stomach secretions.
- Cut back or eliminate chocolate and chocolate-based desserts. The fats and caffeine in chocolate lead to heartburn.
- Try to lose weight. Excess weight squeezes the stomach and forces digestive juices upward. The same happens when you overeat, so instead of eating big lunches and dinners, eat four to six smaller meals spaced out throughout the day.
- Eat slowly.
- Avoid foods or drinks that are excessively hot or cold. Both extremes of temperature will irritate the esophagus.
- If you eat more than usual, loosen your belt after a big meal to keep from squeezing the stomach and forcing acids upward.
- Do not eat a major meal less than four hours before bedtime. The combination of a full stomach and the horizontal resting position will tilt digestive juices the wrong way.
- If you often get heartburn when you lie down, put 6-inch blocks of wood under the bed frame at the head of the bed. This will keep stomach acids from moving into the esophagus.
- If stress causes heartburn, find ways to reduce your stress through professional counseling, relaxation techniques, or regular exercise.

What the Doctor Will Do

As a rule of thumb, if you have to take antacids more than twice a month to relieve heartburn, or if heartburn continues for two weeks, contact your doctor for a checkup. The doctor may take X rays to check for ulcers or a hiatal hernia. He will also go over your daily food intake carefully and may recommend dietary restrictions to counteract heartburn. If you smoke, he will ask you to stop. In some cases, medications will be prescribed to reduce the production of acids in the stomach.

Cause for Concern

Sometimes it's hard to tell the difference between a heart attack and heartburn, especially if chest pain is the *only* symptom. Contact your primary-care physician immediately or go to the nearest hospital Emergency Department if chest pain or pressure lasts more than 2 minutes. You won't die from chest spasms, but heart attacks are the number one killer in this country, and heart damage can often be prevented or minimized if medical care is provided quickly.

Also, one problem with antacids is that their effect is only transient. They buffer acids in the stomach, but if more acid is produced, heartburn could be back in full force in as little as a half hour. Also, frequent use of antacids can mask the heartburnlike pain of stomach ulcers and stomach cancer.

WHAT TO DO

- Don't try to tough heartburn out. Take a dose of an OTC antacid tablet, liquid, or foam. Be aware of possible side effects and interactions with medications.
- Don't drink milk for relief.
- Avoid fat-laden and greasy foods and acidic-drinks. Don't smoke.
- Avoid caffeine.
- Cut back or eliminate chocolate or chocolate-based desserts.
- Lose weight if overweight.
- Don't overeat. Try four to six smaller meals spaced out throughout the day.
- Avoid food or drinks that are excessively hot or cold.
- Place 6-inch blocks of wood under the legs at the head of the bed to keep stomach acids from moving into the esophagus.
- Reduce emotional and physical stress and tension in your life.
- If these conservative measures fail to bring relief, or if you have to take antacids more than twice a month to relieve heartburn, contact your doctor.
- Heart attack and chest pain symptoms are often similar. If chest pain that lasts longer than 2 minutes is your only symptom, contact your primary-care physician immediately or go to the nearest hospital Emergency Department.

HEMORRHOIDS

Samuel B. Labow, M.D.

*Dr. Labow is associate clinical professor of surgery
at North Shore University Hospital–Cornell Medical Center in Long Island, New York*

Hemorrhoids are a common problem, often genetically linked, that are caused by abnormally swollen blood vessels in the rectum and anus as a result of increased pressure from constipation and straining during bowel movements. Hemorrhoids can also result from pregnancy. Signs range from mild discomfort to extreme pain in the rectal area. Bleeding is common in some cases. In addition, bowel movements often become painful, and they may be aggravated from prolonged sitting.

There are two types of hemorrhoids, and they have different symptoms and treatment:

External hemorrhoids are found in and around the anal opening. They are covered by skin and don't bleed. Sometimes in an external hemorrhoid, the blood vessel becomes clotted, which causes the hemorrhoid to swell. This hemorrhoid is often felt as a hard, tender, and very painful bump. These clots develop on their own and are not dangerous or life threatening. Some people, for reasons not understood, are more prone to these painful clots and have to see their doctors as often as every six months for treatment.

In most cases, however, a clotted hemorrhoid is a transitory problem that resolves itself fairly quickly.

The second type are called *internal hemorrhoids,* and are found inside the rectum. The main difference between external and internal hemorrhoids is that when internal hemorrhoids become swollen, they often will bleed.

Blood is typically bright red and appears with or without the trauma or strain of a bowel movement. Sometimes there is a squirting sound as blood goes into the toilet bowl, while at other times a little blood appears on toilet tissue. In severe cases, blood soaks through to the undergarments while one is performing everyday activities.

Treatment

To help ease the pain of a clotted hemorrhoid, soak in a warm bath for 10 to 20 minutes at a time. Continue baths as long as needed.

If the pain doesn't abate within twelve hours, and prevents you from eating, working, or sleeping, then contact your physician.

The doctor will put a local anesthetic into the hemorrhoid to numb it, open the surface of the hemorrhoid and remove the blood clot. No stitches are required, the pain is relieved, and it heals rapidly.

When internal hemorrhoids become large, the pressure of a bowel movement will cause them to protrude out of the rectum and become painful. They will either go back on their own, or will have to be gently pushed back inside. Apply a light coating of petroleum jelly to facilitate the task.

The best treatment and prevention of

hemorrhoids is to produce soft bowel movements. This reduces pressure on the anal area, decreases inflammation, and allows the hemorrhoids to shrink.

This is difficult because the typical American diet lacks enough fiber. Dietary fiber comes from complex carbohydrates —fruits, vegetables, legumes, and whole grains—which the digestive system cannot completely break down. The benefit of these fibers is that they absorb water and create a very soft stool.

Wheat bran, one of the best sources of natural fiber, absorbs water in the colon, increases bulk there by as much as three times, and helps make a stool that is easier to pass. Wheat bran comes in some whole grain breads, or can be added to cereals and other foods.

The target intake of fiber is 15–35 grams a day. To achieve this, gradually begin to eat a variety of fiber-rich foods throughout the day. The reason for the gradual increase is that too much fiber in the digestive system can lead to painful gas, cramping, bloating, and diarrhea.

Besides wheat bran, high sources of fiber include shredded wheat, rolled oats (oatmeal), bran and granola cereals, whole grain breads, kidney and lima beans, corn, potatoes, and peas, brown rice, pasta, prunes, and apples and pears with their skin.

Be sure to drink at least 8 cups of fluid daily. The body needs water to function properly and when water intake is limited, digestion and bowel movements are greatly affected.

Don't sit and read on the toilet for extended periods, and don't strain when you move your bowels. If you're constipated, you will cause hemorrhoids to protrude and make them more prone to irritation and bleeding.

For the pain and itch of hemorrhoids, I don't recommend OTC hemorrhoid remedies. The Food and Drug Administration banned many of these products as of August 1991 because their efficacy and safety couldn't be proved.

The best OTC remedy for hemorrhoids is petroleum jelly. Apply a light coating to the rectum prior to moving your bowels. The petroleum jelly will coat the hemorrhoids and ease the passage of fecal material.

Hygiene plays a major role in reducing symptoms of itching. After each bowel movement, gently clean the anal area with toilet paper. If you have many hemorrhoids, use moistened tissue to make it easier, or else wash with a handcloth and warm, soapy water. Rinse with warm water when you're finished, to remove any irritating soap residue. There are some specially formulated premoistened products available OTC in the pharmacy that can make cleansing easier for some people, but some of these towelettes contain witch hazel, which can be irritating.

A regular exercise program, which can be as basic and simple as walking every day, can provide an effective hemorrhoid treatment. Exercise improves circulation, prevents constipation, and helps prevent hemorrhoids from developing, and aids in the shrinkage of existing hemorrhoids.

Abdominal strain causes increased pressure to rectal/anal veins. When lifting or moving heavy objects, use caution. Lift by bending your knees and pulling up with your arms, straightening your legs simultaneously. For particularly heavy objects, have someone help you.

Standing for long periods may stress the rectal veins. If work requires that you be on your feet, sit or lie down for brief intervals whenever possible.

What the Doctor Will Do

Treatment by a gastroenterologist or colorectal surgeon is necessary when hemorrhoids fail to respond to conservative home therapy, when they bleed persistently, or when pain or itching becomes so intolerable that it interferes with normal activities.

Initial treatment may consist of prescription medications to soothe and reduce pain. If the hemorrhoids don't heal, surgical removal may be recommended.

External hemorrhoids that repeatedly become swollen and painful may require surgery, which is frequently performed in an ambulatory unit, but occasionally may require hospitalization, depending on age and associated medical conditions.

Internal hemorrhoids can be treated with minimal discomfort by a doctor with in-office procedures. Internal hemorrhoids may also be destroyed with sclerotherapy, in which the doctor injects the hemorrhoid with a special chemical. A scar forms and effectively seals off the swollen blood vessel. Some physicians may apply a cold probe and destroy the hemorrhoid by freezing it and causing a scar to form in its place.

Cause for Concern

Laser therapy is touted in many advertisements as the "painless miracle cure" for hemorrhoids. I don't recommend this, however, and see many potential drawbacks. The laser is a powerful instrument with a depth of penetration that may be more than a physician may want.

Lasers are painless when used for internal hemorrhoids, but that's because of the absence of pain fibers inside the rectum. When applied to external hemorrhoids, the laser procedure is every bit as painful as typical surgery. In addition, the area heals slower and is more prone to complications.

Although the presence of blood is a major indicator of an internal hemorrhoid, it can also signal other disorders. At the first sign of blood in your stool, contact your physician for a complete examination. If the blood proves to be from internal hemorrhoids, and if you continue to be troubled by them in the future, make it a point to schedule an annual checkup just to make sure that any bleeding is still hemorrhoid-related.

WHAT TO DO

- Increase fiber intake to 15–35 grams daily and drink 8 cups of liquid a day to produce soft stools.
- Don't strain while defecating.
- Use proper lifting techniques when moving heavy objects.
- Exercise regularly.
- Before a bowel movement, apply a light coating of petroleum jelly to the anus to protect tissue and ease the passage of fecal material.
- Soak in a warm bath for 10–20 minutes.
- At the first sign of rectal bleeding, contact your physician immediately. Rectum, colon, small bowel, and stomach cancers cause bleeding, as do ulcers and

hemorrhoids. Also, contact your physician when hemorrhoids fail to respond to conservative home therapy, when they continue to bleed, or when normal activities are curtailed because of pain, swelling, and itchiness.

HICCUPS

Alan R. Raymond, M.D.

Dr. Raymond is a clinical instructor of Gastroenterology at Beth Israel Medical Center in New York City

Hiccups, or hiccoughs as some people call them, is a mystery ailment with no known purpose. In general, they almost always pass within minutes. In rare cases they may last for a few days.

It's thought that a number of specific nerves in the spinal cord at the back of the neck control hiccups. When something triggers these nerves—eating too quickly, for example—a signal is sent to the phrenic nerve, which controls the diaphragm. The diaphragm signals back to the hiccup center and hiccups begin.

Other triggers of hiccups may be excessive alcohol consumption and smoking. In addition, stress causes a person to subconsciously take in excessive amounts of air, which press up on the diaphragm and stimulate the hiccup center.

Treatment

Although there are dozens, if not hundreds, of hiccup remedies, not one of them is scientifically authenticated. However, some "cures" have been adopted by hiccup sufferers who insist they work. Here are a few:

- Fill a glass with water. Place a metal eating utensil like a knife, fork, or spoon in the water. Sip the water slowly while pressing the handle of the utensil against your temple. By the time the water is finished, the hiccups should vanish.
- Place a teaspoonful of dry granulated sugar on the back of the tongue and then swallow it.
- Fill a glass with ice cubes, add water, stir, and slowly drink. The rapid change of temperature in the esophagus may shut down the hiccup response.
- Hold your breath and count to ten slowly.
- Pull your tongue with your fingers.
- Have someone scare you.
- Stimulate the back of the throat or roof of the mouth with your index finger.
- While sitting, lean forward and compress the chest and diaphragm against the knees.
- Eat dry bread.
- Place a brown paper bag over your nose and mouth, and seal it firmly to your face with your fingers. Rapidly breathe in and out of your mouth ten to fifteen times, and then breathe in the elevated levels of carbon dioxide until the hiccups end.

What the Doctor Will Do

When unrelenting hiccups are not related to any underlying problem, a physician may administer several prescription medications in order to control them. These include prochlorperazine, quinidine, and Dilantin. These drugs have widely different actions, which can act to halt unrelenting hiccups.

Cause for Concern

Several serious underlying diseases are linked with hiccups and should be investigated if your hiccups are persistent, chronic, interfere with work, eating, or sleep, or are associated with weight loss. Lung tumors, pneumonia, gastroesophageal reflux (heartburn), and even a heart attack are often accompanied by hiccups. A chronic case of hiccups may occur as a result of an infection or a tumor in the stomach. Contact your primary-care physician for a complete examination.

WHAT TO DO

- Don't do anything. Be patient and hiccups should stop in a matter of minutes.
- Although not scientifically proved, common self-help remedies may shorten duration of episodes.
- Several serious ailments have hiccups as symptoms. These include pneumonia, heart attack, and certain lung and stomach tumors. If hiccups are chronic, or interfere with work, eating, or sleep, contact your primary-care physician for an examination.

NAUSEA AND VOMITING

Steven Lamm, M.D.

Dr. Lamm is assistant clinical professor of medicine, New York University School of Medicine in New York City

Nausea and vomiting aren't diseases, but symptoms of many conditions such as viral infections, pregnancy, and the smell of toxic chemicals and other odors. Other causes include food poisoning, adverse reactions to different medications, motion sickness, vertigo, severe electrolyte imbalance due to kidney disease or stroke, a blow to the head, increased pressure to the brain from a tumor, diabetes, and severe intestinal obstruction. In most cases, nausea frequently precedes vomiting, which then often relieves the nausea.

In dealing with nausea and vomiting, you have to be in touch with your own body. Ask yourself if this latest condition is a repetition of self-limiting incidents that have occurred in the past. If you don't have high fever or severe abdominal pain along with the nausea and vomiting, you probably need not worry. If the condition is new to you, or persists beyond twenty-four hours, contact your physician.

Treatment

In adults, the most common cause of nausea is a viral gastrointestinal illness. The stomach seems queasy, and the smell of food, sometimes even the thought of it, makes you feel worse. If the major symptom is acute nausea, not accompanied by abdominal pain, vomiting, profuse sweating, or diarrhea, you may have either a viral illness or a form of food poisoning (see FOOD POISONING, page 51). (If people who ate the same contaminated foods as you did, typically meat or mayonnaise-based salad, also have nausea and vomiting, it's probably a form of food poisoning. Contact your co-workers, friends, and family, and then your physician to confirm your suspicion.

If you feel nauseated from some known cause such as a viral infection or motion sickness, vomiting will usually help you feel better. Some people fear vomiting and force themselves not to. Unfortunately, this can greatly intensify the queasy feelings.

Be wary of fluid loss from frequent vomiting and the diarrhea that sometimes accompanies vomiting. Dehydration carries high risk of decreased blood flow to the brain and kidneys. Without upsetting the stomach any further, the key is to replenish lost water and electrolytes, the sodium, potassium, chloride, and bicarbonate elements that are needed by the body in order to function properly.

After you have vomited and no longer feel too nauseated, drink fluids with sugar, including room temperature tea with sugar and honey and noncarbonated ginger ale and cola. Carbonated beverages tend to upset the stomach and can cause vomiting to recur. (To get the fizz out of the soda, shake the container, or leave it with the top off for at least 20 minutes before drinking.)

Sucking on ice cubes or ice chips can be refreshing and give you needed fluids, but you probably won't take in enough liquid this way.

Commercially prepared fluid replacement drinks such as Exceed, Gatorade, and 10K, which are popular with exercisers, can be used to rehydrate.

Take very small sips of your drink. Once you start to gulp the liquid, the stomach becomes distended, and nausea can return. Try to drink at least 6–8 ounces of fluid every hour. A good way to tell if you are getting enough fluids is the frequency and color of your urine. If you urinate frequently and the color is clear or light yellow, you've returned to your normal water balance. Infrequent urination and dark yellow color indicate that you haven't had enough liquids.

Avoid all milk and dairy products for a week to ten days after vomiting. The intestines can't handle milk at this time because the enzyme that metabolizes milk is found on the superficial surface of the intestine. Any gastrointestinal illness destroys this enzyme, reducing the body's ability to digest milk or milk products.

Take liquids only for at least eight hours after vomiting. After that, the stomach should be able to tolerate some solid food. Then I begin what I call the BRAT diet. BRAT is an acronym for bananas, rice, applesauce, and toast.

For electrolyte replacement, eat a banana. This fruit is soft, easy to digest, and provides 500 mg of potassium. Rice provides 160 calories of energy in the form of carbohydrates and is also a little constipating, which is a good thing if you've had diarrhea. Applesauce is easy to digest, provides sugar and some bulk. A slice of toast provides over 100 calories and adds bulk to the stomach.

When going off the diet, let good sense be your guide. Keep portions small and remember to keep drinking fluids with your meals. Temporarily ignore cholesterol considerations and eat a scrambled egg for needed protein. Later, move on to pasta, broth, or tuna, with flavored gelatin for dessert. All of these foods are well tolerated by the stomach.

If you're a milk drinker, it's best to start with skim milk, moving to whole milk a week after all signs of sickness have passed.

For Children

If a child has just vomited and no longer feels nauseated, provide small amounts of clear liquids, such as ginger ale, diluted cola, tea, juice diluted with water, or sugar water. For children under the age of one, prepared electrolyte sugar solutions such as Pedialyte, available OTC in the pharmacy, should be given.

To make sugar water, add 2½ teaspoons of granulated sugar to 1 quart of room temperature water and stir.

Have them sip ½ ounce to 1 ounce every 15 minutes, with the goal of drinking at least 3 ounces every hour. Be careful not to let them fill up, or it could lead to vomiting again. Also, take note if a child says he or she is too sick to drink. If you force children to drink, they may quickly vomit again.

Keep the child on fluids for at least six hours after all feelings of nausea and vomiting have ended. Plain salted crackers can be introduced, followed by small portions of solid easy-to-digest foods such as scrambled eggs, rice, toast, and pasta. As the appetite improves, gradually introduce other foods in the ensuing one to three days.

Do not have the child drink milk until all signs of illness have ended. For an infant whose diet consists primarily of breast milk, continue to breast-feed. If the child is bottle-fed, dilute regular milk portions with half water, and see how it is tolerated. Return to the whole milk diet once vomiting has stopped.

Dehydration brought on by vomiting is a serious problem for infants and toddlers. If the child stops urinating, cries without tears, has a dry mouth, or seems listless, contact your physician.

Cause for Concern

Nausea brought on by gastrointestinal problems normally won't last more than twenty-four hours. If it does, call your doctor. Also, if symptoms seem more severe than you're used to, or if you're older and have other medical problems in which dehydration from vomiting may pose a risk to your health, contact your physician.

If vomit contains bright red blood, it signals bleeding from the esophagus, a symptom of dilated veins often found in alcoholics. Bleeding may also stem from stomach inflammation brought on by aspirin or alcohol. In some cases, bleeding is related to an underlying peptic ulcer. Call your doctor immediately.

Acute abdominal pain is not a symptom of a viral infection. If you have sharp, unremitting stomach pain, it may be stemming from appendicitis, an ulcer, or heartburn. Call your doctor.

A clue that your sickness is something more than viral-induced nausea would be continuous, severe abdominal pain, nausea, and vomiting that lasts more than an hour. This could be a symptom of an intra-abdominal problem of some consequence such as pancreatitis, an obstruction of the intestines by a tumor, or adhesions from prior surgery. Contact your physician immediately.

Also, heart attacks in older people frequently occur with symptoms of nausea and vomiting. Other heart attack symptoms include chest pain or pressure that lasts longer than 2 minutes and radiates to the arms or jaw, heavy sweating, pale skin, and irregular pulse. If you have these symptoms, contact your doctor or get to the nearest hospital Emergency Department.

If your nausea is linked with fever, loss of appetite, headache, and swollen lymph glands in addition to the abdominal pain, contact your physician.

For women, nausea and vomiting in the morning are symptomatic of the first stages of pregnancy. If you haven't had your period for six weeks, contact your gynecologist. Other causes of morning nausea may be related to kidney disease or a reaction to a medication. Contact your physician.

Any nausea and vomiting associated with headaches can be a sign of a migraine headache (see HEADACHE, page 219) or, in rare cases, of a brain tumor. Contact your doctor.

If a headache precedes nausea or vomiting, it may be triggered by intracranial pressure from a tumor or infection. A tip-off here is projectile vomiting. Vomit that shoots out of the mouth is a typical symptom of increased pressure on the brain. Contact your physician immediately.

Various medications will often cause nausea. Cancer drugs, digitalis, megadoses of unprescribed vitamins, codeine cough medicines, theophylline, and various antibiotics are all known to upset the stomach. If you become nauseated after using any of these medicines, contact your physician to discuss other options.

Extremes of emotions can also bring on nausea. Heightened fears and apprehensions upset the stomach and can cause vomiting as well.

Anything that causes decreased vision, such as glaucoma, or brings on pain in the eye can also lead to nausea. Check with your primary-care physician.

WHAT TO DO

- When you feel comfortable enough, try to sip noncarbonated ginger ale or cola, or tea with honey. Young children can be given a sugar-and-water mixture. Adults should drink 6–8 ounces every hour; younger children should drink at least 3 ounces per hour.
- Gradually introduce solid foods over the next one to three days. Follow the BRAT (bananas, rice, applesauce, and toast) diet. Introduce other foods as you feel better.
- Don't drink milk for seven days after a vomiting incident.
- If nausea and vomiting are accompanied by high fever; sharp, unremitting abdominal pain that lasts more than an hour; diarrhea; or sweating, or if the vomiting is unrelenting, contact your doctor immediately or head to the nearest hospital Emergency Department.

Muscles and Joints

GENERAL INFORMATION

When muscles and joints aren't exercised on a regular basis, or if they're overused through vigorous exertion, changes in the bone and surrounding muscle and joints make them prone to injury.

Conditioning the muscles with regular flexibility, strengthening, and aerobic-type activity improves movement and helps prevent common muscle soreness and joint damage.

MUSCULOSKELETAL SPECIALISTS

ORTHOPEDIST (M.D.). An orthopedist is a medical doctor who specializes in the diagnosis, treatment, and prevention of disorders to the musculoskeletal system, including bones, joints, ligaments, tendons, muscles, and nerves. An orthopedist performs surgery when necessary.

OSTEOPATH (D.O.). An osteopath is a trained specialist who can prescribe medication, and also do massage, physical manipulation, and rehabilitation techniques to enhance recovery from injury or disease. Osteopaths are not medical doctors.

PHYSICAL THERAPIST (P.T.). A registered physical therapist is trained to provide techniques and services for aiding recovery and restoring proper movement to the body. In many states, a doctor's prescription is needed for treatment by a physical therapist.

PODIATRIST (D.P.M.). A podiatrist specializes in the diagnosis, treatment, and prevention of foot disorders resulting from injury or disease. A D.P.M. makes independent judgments, prescribes medications, and performs surgery when necessary. Podiatrists are not medical doctors.

continued on page 67

COMMON MUSCULOSKELETAL PROBLEMS

ARTHRITIS
Arthritis is a painful inflammation of one or more joints, with swelling, warmth, redness of overlying skin, pain, and restricted motion the common signs. **Page 68**

CARPAL TUNNEL SYNDROME
A hand disorder that often develops from repetitive finger/wrist flexion, compressing the median nerve to the fingers. If home treatment fails, which it usually does, surgery is necessary to correct the ailment. **Page 72**

LOWER BACK PAIN
This muscle-related condition develops acutely or over time and is often linked to inactivity, poor posture, pregnancy, poor flexibility, hamstring tightness, and a variety of other factors. **Page 73**

MUSCLE CRAMPS
An involuntary, painful, and sustained contraction, typically of the calf or upper leg muscles, usually caused by dehydration, exercising to fatigue, and poor physical conditioning. **Page 83**

MUSCLE SORENESS AND PAIN
A common, self-limiting muscle tear characterized by soreness and pain that occurs with unaccustomed activity, overexertion, or overtraining for sports activity. **Page 78**

SHIN SPLINTS
A muscle or tendon inflammation of the lower leg caused by overstressing the area during exercise, resulting in spasm or diminished blood supply to the leg. Beware: Shin pain may be the first evidence of a stress fracture. **Page 85**

SPRAINS
When a joint is pushed, bent, or twisted beyond its normal range of motion, the ligament that supports the joint is stretched or torn, resulting in pain, inflammation, and swelling. **Page 87**

STIFF NECK

Pain that is felt turning the head, usually caused by degeneration of the neck column or spinal disks, nerve impingement, or neck joint inflammation.

Page 90

TENDINITIS

This inflammation of an overstretched tendon is caused by excessive or improper exercise. Tendons attach muscles to bone.

Page 94

RHEUMATOLOGIST (M.D. or D.O.). Trained as an internal medicine specialist and then in the diagnosis and management of diseases of the joints, ligaments, tendons, and muscles, this doctor treats arthritis, soft tissue conditions such as bursitis, and connective tissue disorders.

ORTHOPEDIC EMERGENCY

DISLOCATION. Disruption of a joint so bone ends are separated and joint no longer functions. Ankle, hip, elbow, shoulder, and fingers are prone to dislocation. Characterized by pain at the joint, swelling,

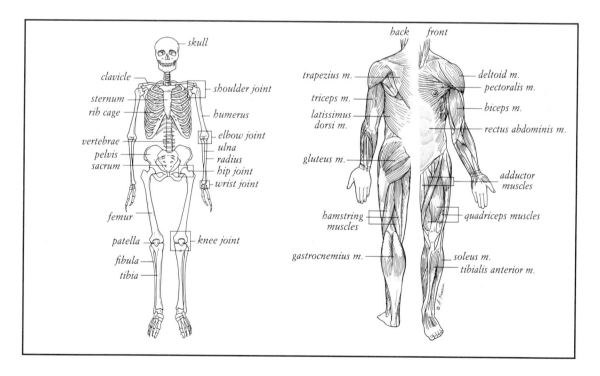

joint deformity, and loss of motion. Protect the damaged area and go to the hospital Emergency Department or contact your physician.

FRACTURE. A break in a bone, ranging from a hairline crack to a severe shattering. Symptoms may include pain, tenderness, swelling, grating sound, and inability to use the injured part. Go to the hospital Emergency Department or contact your physician.

PHYSICIAN'S CARE REQUIRED

GANGLION. A hard nodule of a jelly-like substance that forms in a joint capsule, typically on the back of the wrist or top of the foot. Caused by a mild sprain or defect in joint or tendon sheath. Generally harmless, but doctor may drain or remove it surgically.

HAMMERTOE. A toe deformity, generally the second toe, which causes the toe to become bent and painful. Properly sized shoes or orthoses (corrective appliances) may help relieve pressure, but the condition may require surgery for correction.

OSTEOPOROSIS. Bone deterioration due to poor diet, prolonged immobilization, hormonal disorder, or aging. Doesn't usually produce symptoms, but hip and wrist fractures may occur and low back pain is common with vertebral disintegration. Visible on X ray. Difficult to reverse, but can be helped with regular weight-bearing exercise, calcium, and medication.

ARTHRITIS

Warren Katz, M.D.

Dr. Katz is chairman of the Department of Medicine and chief of the Division of Rheumatology at the Presbyterian Medical Center in Philadelphia, Pennsylvania

Arthritis, a term that means inflammation of the joints, covers over 100 different conditions and it affects one in seven Americans. For reasons still unknown, more than twice as many women as men develop arthritis. Arthritis as a rule attacks between the ages of twenty and sixty, and although symptoms may diminish somewhat with time, it seldom goes away.

Although most forms of arthritis can not be cured, the majority of patients can be made comfortable and functional.

Osteoarthritis

Osteoarthritis, a disease that afflicts more than 16 million Americans, produces symptoms such as mild aching and soreness when moving the weight-bearing joints of the body, especially the hips, knees, or spine. It can also affect the joints at the base of the thumb and big toe. Traumatic injuries to the ankles, shoulder, elbows, or wrists incurred in accidents or from sports participation can also cause osteoarthritis to develop over time.

There is no genetic link to most types of osteoarthritis. By the time we reach the age of sixty, we can all expect to be affected by it to varying degrees. In susceptible individuals, everyday movements eventually wear down cartilage, the smooth cushioning material that covers the ends of skeletal bones that meet to form joints. Once cartilage starts to deteriorate, stiffness and pain result.

To avoid the pain of osteoarthritis, many people move as little as possible. But over a long period of time, this actually causes harm, since the supporting muscles atrophy and even more stress is placed on an injured joint.

Rheumatoid Arthritis

Rheumatoid arthritis, a chronic inflammation of one or many joints of the body, is the second most common form of arthritis. The disease typically attacks joints symmetrically. For example, if your left knee is afflicted, your right knee will become afflicted as well. Prime targets include the elbows, hips, knees, and the small joints of the hands. There is a tendency to deformity and progressive disability.

The exact cause of this disease is unknown. It's suspected that a virus or bacterium somehow triggers the body's immune system to attack its own joints, which then leads to the painful swelling.

A typical case starts when a young to middle-aged woman wakes up and feels a little tired and stiff. Every morning this continues until one morning she notices a joint such as the knee becomes painful, hot to the touch, and a little bit swollen. Days or weeks later, she notices her hands have become painful and stiff and her knuckles have begun to swell.

After a few weeks or months, this woman not only has stiffness and pain in her joints, but has a major disability that interferes with her life.

Treatment

Daily activity such as walking, swimming, or bicycling can at least slow down the development and progression of arthritis. Exercise helps strengthen and maintain overall muscle strength in the body, as well as ligament, tendon, and cartilage health. Physical activity on a daily basis also keeps the joints in proper alignment, which minimizes stress to the weight-bearing joints. In addition, chemical compounds called endorphins are released in the brain during aerobic exercise that help to reduce pain.

The gentle movement of regular exercise is one of the few effective therapies for arthritis. Unfortunately, too many people with arthritis think exercise is harmful or that it aggravates their condition, so they refrain from doing anything.

Before starting any exercise, warm up the muscles first by walking or by performing your exercise at a very slow, controlled pace. Once you begin to perspire lightly and your muscles begin to loosen up, gradually increase the intensity of the exercise. A little shortness of breath is to be expected. Keep all of your movements gentle and smooth.

Exercise for a minimum 20 minutes a

day, three times a week. Whenever you feel joint pain that builds in intensity, ease off or stop completely. It's up to you to know when your exercise is aggravating rather than helping your arthritis symptoms.

The key to success in any exercise program is to find a balance between exercise and adequate rest. Too much or too little of either can worsen your arthritis.

For minor to moderate pain relief, OTC analgesic medication such as aspirin or ibuprofen is excellent. Potential side effects such as nausea can be avoided by taking the medication after meals, or by taking a coated tablet.

Application of heat or ice can provide temporary relief of arthritis pain and soreness. Experiment with both and see which works best for you.

The body works maximally at the normal body temperature of 98.6 degrees F. However, when the body is in pain from arthritis, and you apply extremes of either ice or heat, you can temporarily slow down the transmission of pain nerve impulses to the brain.

To apply ice, fill an ice bag half with water and half with ice cubes. Cover the skin over the tender joint with a towel and apply the ice for 10 minutes. Repeat this three to four times a day. From these brief applications you will get immediate pain relief and feel comfortable. At work, if you don't have access to ice, take a cold can of soda and apply it to the area.

Any form of heat may make your joints feel better when you have arthritis. Take a warm bath or a shower and give this wet heat time to soothe and relax your aching joints. The bathtub is a good place to perform gentle range of motion exercises for your sore joints. For example, if your elbow is sore, slowly bend and straighten it under the water.

Use a whirlpool or swimming pool whenever you get a chance. Moving freely in a large body of water will help to strengthen the muscles and ease the joints through a gentle range of motion.

Another form of wet heat is a hot towel. Heat a hand towel in hot water, wring it out, and place it on your painful joint. *Once the towel cools,* replace it with another and continue this therapy for 20 minutes.

A heating pad can be beneficial when used properly. Don't place the pad directly on the skin. Long applications can cause tissue damage, and mottle the skin. Use heating pads with extreme caution and never use them for more than 20 minutes at a time. Do not sleep on a heating pad.

Touch has a wonderful therapeutic value. Massage your sore joints daily, gently rubbing the muscles around the joint back and forth with the tips of your fingers. Some people like to rub in analgesic liniments purchased OTC because it warms the skin and makes them feel better. There is no evidence that these products relieve soreness, but you may find that by warming the skin, they offer temporary pain relief.

What the Doctor Will Do

Contact your doctor if you develop a persistent pain in any one joint, if you have many painful joints involved at one time, if the pain is causing a disability, or if the pain is associated with fever or diarrhea. Also, seek help if the pain becomes so extreme that you can't sleep.

A primary-care physician can diagnose and treat most arthritis cases. However, if there are complications, you may have to see a rheumatologist or orthopedist.

The specialist will take a detailed history, test the range of motion of the afflicted joints, noting any tenderness, swelling, and deformity. X rays may be taken to check for the presence of arthritis, and a blood test can measure the level of inflammation and help determine the specific cause of the problem. In some cases, stronger anti-inflammatory drugs may be prescribed, and cortisone may be injected directly into the involved joint to reduce inflammation.

If the initial treatment for rheumatoid arthritis doesn't work well, or if the condition worsens, the rheumatologist may use drugs such as gold salts.

As a last resort, a joint destroyed by arthritis may have to be replaced surgically, in order to relieve pain and restore mobility. Because of the limited life-span of the prosthetic devices and the uncertain success of these procedures, a decision to undergo implant surgery must be reached only after careful consideration, consultation with a rheumatologist and orthopedist, and a firm commitment to post-operative rehabilitative physical therapy.

WHAT TO DO

- Take aspirin or ibuprofen according to directions at the first sign of pain or tenderness.
- Perform some form of graded daily activity or exercise to maintain muscle strength and joint stability.
- Warm up properly to loosen muscles and prepare the body for the exercise, and cool down after exercise to keep the blood circulating and reduce chances of lightheadedness and possible muscle soreness.
- Find the right balance between rest and exercise. Too much or too little of each can make arthritis worse.
- Apply hot or cold compresses to sore joints. See which works best for you.
- Perform gentle range-of-motion exercises in the bathtub, whirlpool, or swimming pool.
- Lightly massage the sore areas. Use an analgesic balm if it provides some relief.
- Contact your primary-care physician if you develop a severe or persistent pain in any one joint, if multiple joints are involved, if there is visible inflammation (reddened skin), or the pain is associated with fever, diarrhea, or other generalized symptoms.

CARPAL TUNNEL SYNDROME

A. Griswold Bevin, M.D.

*Dr. Bevin is director of the Hand Rehabilitation Center and chief of the
Division of Plastic Surgery at the University of North Carolina at Chapel Hill*

Carpal tunnel syndrome, or CTS, is a potentially serious hand or wrist disorder usually caused by stressful and repetitive motions of the fingers and wrist. The most common symptom is parasthesia—a feeling that the hand is "asleep."

Other symptoms of CTS may include a burning or tingling sensation in the hand, shooting pain up the forearm, difficulty holding objects, and waking up at night with a tingling, uncomfortable sensation in the hand(s).

The carpal tunnel is a rigid passageway surrounded by bones and ligaments at the wrist. Through it pass the median nerve and eight tendons, the finger flexors. Any repetitive motion that continues for extended periods, such as playing the drums, lifting weights, sorting mail, typing on a desktop computer or video display terminal, paddling a canoe, playing the piano, or doing carpentry may cause the sheaths covering the tendons to become inflamed and swollen. This may compress the median nerve against the confines of the carpal tunnel, causing CTS.

This syndrome can also occur during the latter months of pregnancy, with thyroid problems, diabetes, use of certain birth-control medications, a fractured wrist bone, or arthritis.

CTS is more prevalent today because of the use of devices that allow and/or require repetitive finger motion. Also, advanced technology divides jobs into ever smaller tasks, and workers make fewer motions more frequently.

CTS is at least twice as common among women, probably because they traditionally have worked as typists and keyboard operators, and now even more are employed in computer work.

I've had CTS off and on for a few years now. It's related to the repetitive flexion of my fingers at my weekend hobby of working on my cars, and taking care of our gardens and woods. During the weekend, numbness and tingling develops across the thumb, index, and long fingers, and sometimes half of my ring finger. It doesn't affect my little finger. The discomfort comes and goes, sometimes even awakens me at night, but clears up in a day and doesn't interfere with my surgical practice. Eventually, I will need surgery to correct the problem.

When CTS flares and bothers me, I may rub my fingers together or shake my hands to relieve the tingling.

Treatment

If you think you have CTS, see your physician or a doctor who specializes in the hand. If your condition is mild, there are several things you can do in an effort to relieve the pressure on the wrist. If successful, you may be able to avoid surgery. However, home treatment fails nearly all of the time.

Splinting the wrist with a brace can be helpful, but only when the brace keeps your wrist *and* fingers from flexing. Your doctor will suggest the proper brace and where to purchase one.

Anti-inflammatory medication such as aspirin or ibuprofen taken after eating may help relieve CTS discomfort and inflammation in some people. However, there is no scientific evidence that it does.

Vitamin B_6 may be helpful and effective in treating CTS and has been slightly helpful in my case. Take 100 mg twice daily. Vitamin B_6 is inexpensive and quite harmless at this dosage. However, *never* exceed this dosage.

What the Doctor Will Do

If the pins-and-needles sensation of CTS continues after two months of this conservative home treatment, contact your physician for another examination. The doctor may recommend a nerve conduction test to check the ability of the median nerve to transmit impulses. If surgery is necessary, it is usually a rather short operation done in an outpatient setting. Complete recovery requires three to six weeks, and most people are able to return to their regular employment.

WHAT TO DO

- Wear a special brace to keep your wrist *and* fingers from flexing.
- Take anti-inflammatory medications such as aspirin or ibuprofen.
- Take 100 mgs of vitamin B_6 twice daily. *Never* exceed this dosage.
- If the pins-and-needles sensation continues after two months, contact your doctor for another exam. Further testing is needed, and surgery may be in order.

LOWER BACK PAIN

Peter A. Moscovitz, M.D.

Dr. Moscovitz is associate clinical professor of Orthopedic Surgery at George Washington University and consulting Spine Surgeon at the George Washington University Spine Center in Washington, D.C.

Eighty percent of all Americans will suffer from lower back pain at some time in their lives. Backaches cause more lost work time than any other physical ailment, with the exception of the common cold.

Back pain may be caused by a number of underlying problems such as arthritis, bone spurs, or deformities, either inborn or acquired. Still, 90 percent of all lower back pain is caused by muscle or joint injuries related to some form of overuse. Overuse may be sudden, as in picking up a heavy box, or cumulative, as in beginning an exercise program.

Back injuries are often made worse by

tension and stress, or posture, a sedentary life-style, obesity, pregnancy, a sagging mattress, sleeping on your stomach, and poor body mechanics—you lifted that box improperly. In some cases, but not all, the pain is caused by rupture or tear of a spinal disk. However, probably no more than 2 percent of all back problems can be helped by surgery.

When you first develop lower back pain, don't do anything for your back until you have personalized your problem and come up with some answers. Ask yourself the following series of questions: What happened? What was I doing yesterday? What did I just do two seconds ago? Is this related to some problem I have had in the past? Does it feel different from the last time my back hurt?

Also, ask yourself what it is that hurts in particular. Take stock of the situation and pinpoint where the pain is. Is it my back or buttocks? Is it my leg? Does pain go all the way to my feet? What are the unusual or funny sensations that I feel?

You also need to ask yourself what makes the back pain feel worse. If you roll over and try to get out of bed, is it worse? Is it worse if you stretch your legs out? When you turn or twist, does the pain seem worse?

Try to find what makes the pain lessen. If you draw your knees up, if you stretch out, if you get out of bed and walk around, does it make the lower back feel better? These self-tests may be reasonable trials because sometimes back pain is better if you get up and move around, and the sooner you do it, the better you will feel. Would you feel better if you got into a hot tub, put a heating pad on the back, or used an ice pack? These are individual experiments you need to carry out. See how you feel after trying them, and then go from there.

On the other hand, you may also find that it's absolutely necessary to lie very still and try to adjust your position so you minimize the pain and get some relief.

Remember that 90 percent of lower back pain gets better with simple, conservative care. Sometimes it may take three weeks, but it eventually gets better. Many of the people who fall into the 10 percent who don't get better within three to six weeks will get better over time without major invasive treatment like injections or surgery.

It's often a bitter pill to swallow when you find that you may have to miss work for a while, that you may not be able to dance, or that sexual activity will be tricky for some time. Be reassured that most people with lower back pain do get better within three to six weeks, and most feel better within the first forty-eight to seventy-two hours.

Treatment

When you develop lower back pain, there are several things you can do to help relieve it. Start with the basic lower back care program described here. If that doesn't work within forty-eight to seventy-two hours, contact your physician. If your back is improving, even slightly, then keep up what you are doing.

BED REST. Bed rest for twenty-four to forty-eight hours after the onset of severe lower back pain is helpful, because it reduces inflammation and irritation of the muscles. Lie on your side with your knees drawn up slightly toward your chest with a pillow between your knees. Other options include lying on your back with two or more pillows under your knees and no more than one pillow under your head, or lying on your stomach with a pillow directly under your hips and one under your ankles. If you have kyphosis, an excessive outward curvature of the spine causing you to become round-shouldered, you may feel more comfortable lying on your side with several pillows under your head.

Most people find forty-eight hours of rest is needed to relieve back pain, though some may require less. The rule of thumb is to let your pain be your guide. If you can't straighten up, remain in bed. But if you can stand for periods of time before the pain becomes too intense, then do so. Studies show that two days of bed rest is sufficient in most cases of lower back pain, and is often as effective as seven days of bed rest. Actually, the sooner you can get out of bed and start the back exercises to stretch and strengthen your sore muscles, the better you'll feel.

POSITION. If you develop lower back pain after lifting a heavy object, or if you just wake up and it's there, lie on the floor on your back with your knees bent and your feet flat on the floor. Slowly pull your knees up to your chest, if possible, to aid further in relaxing the back muscles and breaking some of the spasm. Hold this position for five minutes.

Another position that might offer pain relief is to lie with your back flat on the floor. Raise your legs up to the seat of a chair, or have someone lift them up for you, and let your calf muscles lie across the seat of the chair. Rest in this position for 5 minutes.

ICE AND HEAT. If you feel soreness in one specific area of the lower back, put an ice pack directly on it. The ice mini-mizes swelling and slows down, blocks, or temporarily stops the transmission of pain messages to the brain. To avoid damaging the skin, wrap the ice in a towel. Remove the ice when it begins to hurt, generally within 5 minutes or so. Repeat the ice procedure 10 to 15 minutes later. Don't keep the ice on the back longer than 30 minutes at a time or the back muscles may become chilled, which can lead to more muscle spasm. (A good way to apply the ice is to fill paper cups with water, freeze them, then tear away the top portion to expose the ice, and gently massage the skin with it.) Another technique is to apply a frozen bag of rice or beans to your lower back. Put the bag back in the freezer until needed again. You can cook the contents when you feel better.

During the first twenty-four hours, continue with the ice treatment in two sessions lasting no more than two hours each of the on-and-off application.

Heat may provide better pain relief for you than ice. In some cases of chronic lower back pain, hot compresses applied with a hot water bottle, a heating pad, or a towel heated in water can help relieve spasm symptoms after the first twenty-four hours. Whichever heating method you use, keep the heat on the lower back for upward of a half hour and reapply it up to four times a day. But be careful. Scalding can occur.

A hot bath or shower or sitting in a hot tub will also increase blood flow to the lower back area and bring some welcome pain relief. A note of caution: Since the hot water dilates the blood vessels so dramatically, lightheadedness may develop, and you can easily fall getting out of the tub or shower. End your session with tepid water to prevent this.

MEDICATION. Aspirin and ibuprofen are good pain relievers and serve as anti-inflammatories. Prescription anti-inflammatory medications have not been proved to offer significant improvement over them. Therefore, if you don't have high blood pressure, stomach trouble, liver or kidney disease, take either buffered aspirin or ibuprofen with meals according to dosage recommended on the label. These drugs often help reverse back pain quickly. Acetaminophen (Tylenol) is a third choice for lower back pain. Although it lacks anti-inflammatory properties, it may provide sufficient pain relief.

As a word of caution when your back is in spasm: Only travel if it's an absolute necessity. Take all meals in bed or while standing up. Avoid sitting. This increases strain on the back. Also, remember that back pain will interfere with activities that typically make up your daily living schedule. Work will be disrupted, you may not be able to interact socially or even perform simple tasks. Note, too, that this injury may predispose you to temporary feelings of depression, anger, or melancholy. It is good to have someone you can share these feelings with.

BACK EXERCISES. Once you are relatively pain-free, begin exercises that will gently stretch and strengthen your muscles. Perform the following four exercises in the morning and again at night on a carpeted floor. Do them slowly and without tugging or bouncing.

Pelvic tilt. Lie on your back with your knees bent at a 45 degree angle, your feet flat on the floor, and your arms at your sides. Relax and concentrate on your breathing. As you inhale, contract your buttock muscles as well as your abdominal muscles as tightly as you can. As you do this, you will feel your lower back flatten against the floor. Count slowly to 5 and then relax the muscles.

Lower back stretch. Lie on your back on the floor with your knees bent at a 45 degree angle, feet flat on the floor, and arms comfortably at your sides. Grab your right knee with two hands and slowly pull it toward your right shoulder as far as it can comfortably go. Don't jerk or tug your leg or raise your head off the floor. Don't let your lower back rise up from the floor. Hold the leg for the count of 10 and then slowly return the foot to the floor. Repeat the same movement with the left leg.

Repeat the right-leg-left-leg cycle five times, and when your back feels stronger, increase to ten repetitions.

Double knee raise. Start with knees raised, feet on the floor. Grab your knees with both hands and gently pull them toward the shoulders. Once you have pulled them as far as possible, roll your head up slowly toward your knees, hold for the count of 10, and then slowly return to the floor. Repeat this stretch five times.

Partial sit-up. Lie on the floor on your back with your knees bent at a 45 degree angle and feet flat on the floor. Keep your arms folded across your chest. Tuck your chin in toward your chest, tense your buttock and abdominal muscles, and gradually raise your shoulders off the floor as you exhale, aiming your elbows to your thighs. Hold this position for the count of 5 and slowly return to the floor. Repeat for a total of five to ten times.

I experienced severe back pain many years ago after falling 20 feet from a ski lift, and I still perform these and other lower back exercises intermittently in order to maintain control over my back. One thing you must understand about lower back pain is that once you've injured your back and have recovered, you are *not* necessarily cured of a lower back problem, you have only controlled it. A healed lower back injury may not return the anatomy and mechanical function of the back to normal. You still need to perform the stretching and strengthening exercises to prevent a recurrence.

Prevention

- Sit up straight in your chair because slouching puts additional stress on the spine and back muscles.
- Lift heavy objects by bending the knees first and making the legs, not the back, lift the load.
- Use a firm mattress for adequate back support. Sleep on your side or back because sleeping on your stomach can increase stress on the joints of the lower back.
- Participate in a regular fitness program designed to build and maintain cardio-respiratory fitness as well as muscular strength, flexibility, and stamina.
- If you have a back problem, avoid activities that require twisting, lifting, or bending. These can include weight lifting, golf, and tennis. If such activities are important to you, be mindful of the risks and don't overdo.
- Low-impact activities such as walking, ballroom dancing, swimming, water aerobics, cross-country skiing, in-line skating, light jogging, and bicycling help with weight control, reduce tension, and provide good physical fitness. Consult with your physician before beginning any new fitness program.

Cause for Concern

If you have back pain, or have some problem that you think may relate to your back, and you also have trouble controlling your bowel or bladder, contact your physician immediately. This is a medical emergency.

Your family physician should be called whenever you have concerns about any type of lower back pain. In some instances, specialists in the field of orthopedic surgery, physiatry (prevention of disease by means of physical agents), neurosurgery, neurology, or rheumatology might be suitable consultants if needed. You should also contact the doctor if you have four to five days of unremitting pain in the lower back, especially if it awakens you from sleep at night, if acute pain develops for no apparent reason and doesn't go away within twenty-four hours, if you develop pain or numbness or have tingling sensations that move down your leg, or whenever you suffer back pain from a fall, car crash, or other type of traumatic accident.

What the Doctor Will Do

- The doctor will take a detailed history, and perform a complete physical exam to check reflexes and to rule out more serious disk or nerve problems.
- In some cases, your doctor may refer you to an orthopedist for further examination.

WHAT TO DO

- Lie immediately on your back on the floor with your knees bent and your feet flat on the floor. Hold this position for 5 minutes.

- Apply ice to the sore area. After twenty-four to forty-eight hours, apply heat compresses if you find it brings relief.
- Take buffered aspirin, ibuprofen, or acetaminophen.
- Rest in bed if pain is severe.
- Lie on your side in bed with knees drawn up slightly toward your chest and a pillow between your knees.
- Take all meals in bed or while standing.
- Avoid sitting.
- Begin stretch and strengthening exercises once your back is no longer in spasm and you are relatively pain-free.
- Contact your family physician when you have concerns about lower back pain. Call immediately if you have bowel or bladder problems. Also, call if you have four days of unremitting lower back pain, if acute pain develops for no apparent reason and doesn't go away within twenty-four hours, if you develop numbness or have a tingling sensation in your leg, or whenever you develop back pain after a fall or car accident.

MUSCLE SORENESS AND PAIN

Harlen C. Hunter, D.O.

Dr. Hunter is director of the St. Louis Orthopedic Sports Medicine Clinic in Chesterfield, Missouri

Go out for a weekend run after six days of inactivity, carry a 50-pound bag of peatmoss from your car to the garden, or chop a cord of firewood. Within twenty-four to forty-eight hours after performing any of these strenuous activities, your muscles will feel sore and stiff, and they can remain that way for up to a week or more. This muscle soreness, called delayed-onset muscle soreness, or DOMS, is due to microscopic muscle damage caused by vigorous physical activity.

Another form of muscle pain and soreness is a muscle strain, a more serious problem that's commonly known as a "pulled muscle." Muscle strain results from suddenly overstretching a muscle through excessive stress or prolonged use, which causes the muscle to tear and eventually contract. Muscle strains are common among sedentary people who try to do something very active such as running down the street to catch a taxi, or lifting something way beyond their strength. Strains are also common among trained athletes who neglect their warm-up prior to a workout or competition.

The most common sites of muscle strain are where a muscle stretches between two joints, such as the biceps muscle that connects the shoulder to the elbow, or the hamstring, which runs from the hip to the knee.

Symptoms, which vary from mild to moderate, as a rule develop immediately and worsen over time. They include localized pain, tenderness, and in some cases swelling.

Treatment

For symptomatic relief from muscle soreness and strain, there are several things you can do:

Take a warm shower, or bath, use a heating pad, or whirlpool if you have access to one. The heat helps push out cellular debris in the muscles.

Remain active, if possible. Actually, a very light repetition of the same or similar activity that brought on the soreness will help loosen your muscles and force out the inflammatory fluids without further injuring the muscles.

Many people with sore muscles rub OTC liniments on them. These liniments create a feeling of warmth to the skin by dilating surface blood vessels. However, liniments don't penetrate deeply enough through either the skin or the fat layer above the muscles to improve soreness, and therefore don't promote healing.

However, when you vigorously massage a liniment over sore muscles, it's not the liniment that helps, but rather the act of massaging. This stimulates circulation and temporarily relieves soreness.

Don't take aspirin when your muscles are sore. Aspirin thins the blood, and whenever you have overexercised and caused a breakdown of the muscles, aspirin will cause you to bleed more easily, prolonging recovery. Take acetaminophen if you feel the need of a pain reliever.

If you have a mild to moderately strained muscle, apply ICE techniques immediately to help promote recovery. This means using *ice, compression,* and *elevation.* In the case of soreness and pain, you should not rest the affected muscle as you would do for more serious conditions.

Muscle strain has to be treated quickly to reduce swelling, so apply ice immediately to the damaged muscle. If you have ice cubes in a bag, place a thin cloth under the bag to prevent superficial frostbite. If you are using crushed ice in a plastic bag, apply it directly to the skin because the melting water will form a protective barrier to prevent skin damage.

Let pain be your guide when determining how long to use ice. Once the area starts to ache from the ice treatment and you feel an unbearable discomfort, remove the ice. Then, when the pain from the muscle strain comes on again, put the ice back on and leave it there until the ice causes intense discomfort again. Repeat this procedure as often as possible throughout the day.

Also take an anti-inflammatory medication such as ibuprofen within the first half hour after straining a muscle. This helps reduce swelling.

After applying ice, wrap an elastic athletic bandage around the muscle to compress it, prevent swelling, and provide additional support. Wrap from the tip of the extremity toward the trunk, putting just a gentle tension on the bandage as you wrap.

Elevate the strained muscle higher than your heart to drain any accumulated fluids out of the area. If necessary, prop up the injured body part on pillows to keep it elevated.

When swelling disappears—generally twenty-four to forty-eight hours later—stop the cold treatment and switch to heat therapy. Take a bath or shower in 100 degree F water for 20 minutes. The heat increases blood flow and brings in white blood cells to help clear out any molecular debris. Return to the heat two hours later for another 20-minute session.

Don't remain completely inactive during this recovery period. Once swelling has stopped and pain diminished, in the case of a leg injury for example, I like a person to start walking or even begin mild jogging at an intensity just under their threshold of pain. This gentle activity helps to keep the damaged leg muscle from shortening and prevents scar tissue from forming in the area.

Once there is no pain at all in the muscle, begin a gentle stretching program to get back your normal range of motion. Start a muscle strengthening program and then gradually resume your normal exercise routine.

Prevention

Muscle soreness, and even torn muscles, typically develop when you overexert untrained muscles. Anything from household chores to a vigorous tennis match can cause a problem. The following is the best program for preventing muscle soreness and strain from occurring in the future:

- Begin a gradual training program that emphasizes gentle flexibility exercises, muscle strengthening, and low-intensity aerobic exercise.
- Gradually increase this program's intensity over a period of weeks.
- Flexibility returns the full range of motion to your joints, relieves everyday muscle tension, keeps the muscles supple, promotes circulation, and prepares you for a full array of injury-free activities.
- Stretching promotes flexibility. The best time to stretch is to take 5 to 10 minutes out of your day to do it, such as on lunch break, or at home after work.

MINI STRETCHING AND STRENGTHENING PROGRAM

When you stretch, don't bounce or force your muscles to go farther than they can. Stretch to the point of easy tension, relax, hold it for up to 30 seconds and then stop. If you feel any pain, ease off until the pain goes away, or else stop the stretch immediately. Anytime there is pain, it means you're pushing too hard.

On the lower body, focus on stretching the major muscles, which include the hamstring and quadricep muscles on the back and front of the thigh, the calf muscles on the back of the shin, and the lower back area. For the upper body, stretch the shoulders and upper back.

Incorporate the following basic stretches into your daily routine. Hold each stretch for up to 30 seconds and repeat each exercise four times, twice daily.

HAMSTRINGS. Stand in front of a desk or table, and with one foot on the ground and pointed straight ahead, raise your opposite foot up and onto the edge of the desk. Bend at the knee and gently lean forward to stretch the hamstrings.

QUADRICEPS. Stand facing away from a desk, table, or fence, and raise one leg up behind you and rest the top of your foot there. Gently begin to pull with your foot as if you were trying to kick down with your leg. This will stretch the quadriceps on the front of your leg. For safety, hold on to a chair for balance while doing this stretch.

CALVES. Stand with your hands on your hips, both feet flat on the floor, one foot behind and the other foot in front, with the knee in front slightly flexed. Keep the back leg straight and lean forward until a stretch is felt in the back of the rear leg. Hold this position steady and *do not* bounce.

LOWER BACK. With your feet shoulder-width apart and knees slightly bent, slowly bend forward at the waist with your arms hanging comfortably at your sides. The longer you hold the stretch, the more your hamstrings and lower back will loosen and your hands will begin to descend closer toward the floor.

SHOULDERS. Sitting, hold your arms straight out in front and then swing them horizontally to the left as far as possible and then swing back to the right. Movement should not be jerky, but slow and controlled.

UPPER BACK. Sitting in a chair, interlace your fingers together behind your head and flare your elbows straight out at the sides. Slowly try to bring your shoulder blades together; when you feel the tension, hold the stretch for 20 seconds.

To build muscular strength and endurance without having to spend any money on exercise equipment or health club memberships, you can use the resistance of your own body by performing push-ups, sit-backs, and wall squats in the privacy of your own home.

PUSH-UPS. Push-ups are a perfect exercise because they not only strengthen the shoulders and arms, but also your abdominal muscles. The key here is proper form.

Lie face-down on the floor with your palms flat on the floor a little wider than shoulder width, feet close together, legs out straight. Push up off the floor with your hands and then return to the ground, barely touching your chest, before pushing up again. Keep your back straight as you descend and don't rush the push-up. You're not trying to see how many you can do, but how many you can perform properly before tiring.

Abdominal strength is the key to a strong back and powerful athletic movement. Most people are lacking here, especially those who have been inactive for a long time. This is where sit-backs will be a great help in firming up abdominal strength.

SIT-BACKS. Start by sitting on the floor with your knees raised, feet flat on the ground. Cross your arms over your chest and slowly lower yourself back toward the floor. Once your shoulders touch, push yourself back to the sitting position with your elbows and repeat the drill. Do five repetitions, and add one more each day.

WALL SQUATS. Wall squats will develop the leg strength in your thighs and buttocks needed for most sports. Start with your back to the wall, feet flat on the ground. Gradually lower yourself down until your knees are at a 90 degree angle. If you have knee pain, raise yourself up higher. Hold the position for 20 seconds, come up for 20 seconds to rest, and then repeat the drill five times. After several sessions, increase your time to 30 seconds on, 30 seconds off.

WALKING. Walking is the easiest way to improve cardiovascular strength and endurance, and is also the safest way to ease yourself gradually into a more demanding exercise program. Start by trying to walk for 15–20 minutes a day and continue at this level for about a month. As you progress, vary both your routes and speeds to keep the walk interesting and challenging.

After a month of regular walking, you have laid the muscular and cardiovascular groundwork and are prepared to start light jogging if you so desire. Start by walking for 2 minutes, then jog for 1 minute. Continue this walk/jog routine for 20 minutes.

The next week, walk for 1½ minutes and jog for 1½ minutes, continuing this routine for 20 minutes.

On the third week, walk 1 minute, then run for 2 minutes for a total of 20 minutes. By week four, run nonstop for 20 minutes, and each week thereafter increase your distance covered by a quarter of a mile.

What the Doctor Will Do

If you have muscle soreness that won't go away after five days of home measures, or if you feel a "pop" or snap of a muscle while performing some activity, contact your primary-care physician. The doctor will take a history and perform a physical examination. If needed, he may tape the area to provide extra support, prescribe more powerful pain relievers and anti-inflammatory medication, or prescribe a course of physical therapy.

Cause for Concern

In severe cases, the muscle may rupture and tear completely. Symptoms include immediate and severe pain, an inability to move the muscle normally, swelling, with a distinct bulge at the pain site, and a black and blue discoloration around the injury. Contact your physician immediately if you rupture your muscle.

WHAT TO DO

For muscle soreness:
- Take a warm shower, bath, or whirlpool.
- Perform a light repetition of the same activity that initially brought on the soreness.
- Massage your sore muscles.
- Take acetaminophen if you feel the need for a pain reliever.

A muscle strain is a common injury that results from suddenly overstretching a muscle, causing tissue damage, a torn or ruptured muscle, and contraction. To minimize symptoms of pain, tenderness, and swelling:
- Apply ice immediately to the damaged muscle.
- Take anti-inflammatory medication such as ibuprofen within the first half hour.
- Wrap an elastic athletic bandage around the muscle to compress it and provide support.
- Elevate the strained muscle higher than your heart.
- When swelling has stopped, switch to heat therapy.
- Begin a gentle stretching program to get back normal range of motion when pain and swelling are gone.
- Start a muscle strengthening program.
- If you have muscle soreness that won't go away after five days of home therapy, or if you suddenly feel a snap or pop in a muscle and experience severe pain, contact your physician.

MUSCLE CRAMPS

Richard Levandowski, M.D.

Dr. Levandowski is director of Primary Care, Sports Medicine, and clinical associate professor of the Department of Family Medicine, University of Medicine and Dentistry of New Jersey–Robert Wood Johnson Medical School in New Brunswick, New Jersey

A muscle cramp can occur anywhere in your body, although the calf and thigh muscles are the most common sites. No one has yet pinpointed the exact cause of cramps, but it's thought that a number of factors may be at work, including dehydration, electrolyte (sodium and potassium) imbalance in the blood, poor physical conditioning, exercising to fatigue, or an improper diet.

Muscle cramps occur more often in people who exercise regularly. Athletic-minded people often sweat profusely or are on low-salt diets, and the cramping may be related to that.

Prevention

- Adequate hydration is perhaps the most important way to prevent cramping. Drink a minimum of a half-gallon of liquid (eight 8-ounce glassfuls) throughout the day.
- Water is the best liquid to drink. Nonalcoholic drinks such as juice, decaffeinated tea or coffee (caffeine causes dehydration), lemonade, soft drinks, seltzer, prepared sports drinks such as Gatorade, and soup also help you meet your water quota.
- Drink before you are thirsty. Thirst is not an adequate indicator of how much water the body needs because the brain first reacts to the level of salt concentration in the blood before it recognizes fluid loss.
- Drink at least 20 ounces of water (2½ cups) one hour before exercising. Take a water bottle with you whenever you exercise. As you work out, drink 4–6 ounces of water (½ to ¾ cup) every 12 to 15 minutes.
- Weigh yourself before and after exercising. A postworkout weight loss of 2 pounds may often be a sign of dehydration. To recover weight lost after exercise, drink at least 16 ounces of water (2 cups) for each pound lost.
- Stretching techniques used before and after exercise help prevent most cramps. If you are prone to leg cramps, gently stretch out the calf muscles by doing wall push-ups. (To perform a wall push-up, stand 4 feet away from a wall with your feet flat on the ground, legs straight. Don't bend your knees. Bending your elbows, lean into the wall and support yourself with your hands. Hold the stretch for 10 seconds, push back up, and then repeat.)
- To stop nocturnal cramping, keep sheets and blankets tucked in loosely to take pressure off your legs. In some chronic cases of leg cramps, quinine sulfate tablets may be prescribed by your doctor and taken at bedtime as a preventive measure.

Treatment

For quick relief from a muscle cramp, stretch the muscle out. For example, if your hamstring suddenly cramps, extend your leg straight out, thereby stretching the quadriceps and hamstring muscles. This stretch should cause the hamstring to relax. Massage the area with your fingers.

For a cramped calf muscle, sit on the floor with your leg outstretched. Grab your toes and pull the foot back by the toes in the direction of your face. Once the calf cramp stops, massage the area with your fingers.

If the stretching and massage relieve the cramp, it is generally safe to return to exercise. However, if the cramp recurs, stop exercising, stretch out the cramp, and drink plenty of fluids. Continuing to exercise may lead to a muscle strain.

For extreme or prolonged cramps, apply ice directly to the cramped muscle. This causes the muscle to relax and should stop the pain. An athletic trainer's trick for calf cramps is to take your shoe off and put an ice pack to the sole of the foot. In lieu of an ice pack, put the foot directly into a bucket of ice or ice water.

While your leg muscle is in spasm, try this unusual but often effective cramp treatment. Pinch the upper lip just below the nose with the thumb and forefinger as hard as possible. Many times the cramp will dissipate or even stop.

Although many people assume a nutritional deficiency causes muscle cramps, that's usually not the case. Factors such as overexercise, fatigue, poor conditioning, and water loss should first be eliminated before you look for a nutritional deficiency.

If you drink enough water but still cramp, add more salt to your food and increase the amount of potassium in the diet as well. Add salt in cooking, sprinkle it on food, or else eat salt-rich snacks such as pretzels or crackers to help restore any electrolyte imbalance in the body. If you have heart disease or take any medications, contact your physician first. Do not take salt tablets. Salt tablets cause excessive amounts of water to be drawn into the stomach, which can cause dehydration, nausea, and vomiting.

To increase the amount of potassium in your daily diet, eat potassium-rich foods such as bananas, tomatoes, raisins, apricots, or melons, or drink a glass of tomato, pineapple, or orange juice.

Cause for Concern

If you are still bothered by muscle cramps after trying these methods, or if you experience cramping or muscle spasms in the lower back or neck, accompanied with pain that goes down the leg or into the arm, contact your physician.

WHAT TO DO

To avoid or relax painful cramps:
- Drink a minimum of a half-gallon of liquid, spaced throughout the day.
- Drink before you become thirsty.
- Drink at least 20 ounces of water (2½ cups) one hour before exercising. As you work out, drink 4–6 ounces of water (½–¾ cup) every 12 to 15 minutes.
- Drink at least 16 ounces of water (2 cups) for each pound lost due to exercise.
- Stretch the cramped muscle for quick relief.

- Stretch before and after exercise.
- Apply ice directly to a cramped muscle.
- Pinch the upper lip as hard as possible to relieve leg cramps.
- Keep sheets and blankets loose to prevent nocturnal leg cramping.
- Add more salt to your food and increase the amount of potassium in the diet if the above methods don't help prevent cramps.
- Contact your physician if you are still bothered by muscle cramps, or if you experience cramping in the lower back or neck that is accompanied with pain that radiates down the leg or into the arm.

SHIN SPLINTS

Lyle J. Micheli, M.D.

Dr. Micheli is associate clinical professor of Orthopedic Surgery at Harvard Medical School and director of Sports Medicine at Children's Hospital in Boston, Massachusetts

Shin splints, an inflammation of tendons and muscles of the shin, is typically brought on by the impact forces of exercise.

The shin bone, or tibia, is covered by the periosteum, a band of soft tissue that has both nerve tissue and a blood supply. Just above the ankle and below the knee, tendons help attach muscles to the periosteum. However, when the shin is overstressed, problems can develop in the periosteum, in the tendons, on the shin bone, in the muscle, or in the four muscle compartments of the lower leg covered with a wall of connective tissue called fascia. If recurrent, this latter condition is called chronic compartment syndrome.

Shin splints are a common, often seasonal injury that usually occur when you start to run after a long layoff. They can also come from playing a sport such as tennis on a hard surface, when you change your workout shoes to a different model, when you dramatically increase your workouts, or when you put on a substantial amount of weight and begin to exercise.

Anterior shin splint is due to an injury to muscles or tendons that help lift the front of the foot, and results in pain and tenderness on the front outside of the leg. Posterior pain, a soreness that radiates along the back and inner side of the lower leg or ankle, is typically caused by stressed muscles that help support and stabilize the arch of the foot.

A stress fracture, a small hairline crack in the shin bone, develops slowly after repeated stress and impact to the legs. Symptoms develop during exercise and include a sudden, burning pain.

Unlike other forms of shin splints, where pain is spread out over the shin, you can pinpoint the spot from which the pain of a stress fracture is emanating. In mild to moderate cases, the pain subsides when exercise ends and will heal completely with adequate rest of a month or more.

Treatment

At the first sign of pain in the shins, stop your activity. Trying to exercise through the soreness will only aggravate the condition and cause it to worsen.

Immediately massage the area with ice to reduce inflammation and irritation. The ice acts like a quick-acting, anti-inflammatory medication. The best way to ice is to take a paper cup, fill it with water, and leave it in the freezer. When it's frozen, tear off a small portion from the top to expose the ice and then massage the sore area for 20 minutes. Repeat this four times a day.

For pain relief and help to decrease the swelling, take 2 ibuprofen tablets three times daily.

Don't apply heat to the area. Shin splints are an inflammatory condition, and heat will only irritate the area even more.

Healing time can be as little as two to three weeks if you cut back on your exercise and begin aggressive self-help measures, but in some severe cases recovery can take as long as twelve to fourteen weeks before pain subsides.

Total inactivity is definitely not the answer to shin splints. Once you resume training after the problem has gone, you've lost a good deal of conditioning, and shin splints can recur while you are trying to make up for lost time. A way around this is to perform an exercise that doesn't involve foot impact. This can include swimming, water aerobics or water running, in-line skating, cross-country skiing, bicycling, and stair climbing. These workouts will help elevate your heart rate and promote aerobic fitness, but without stressing your shins.

Once you switch your land workouts to the water, you'll be amazed at the results. Take a tip from many world-class athletes, and begin water running workouts to help maintain your conditioning.

If you don't know how to swim or have difficulty staying afloat, use a special flotation device such as a Wet Vest or Aqua-Jogger (for information, call 1–800–922–9544) to keep your head above water and provide proper buoyancy. Forty minutes of water exercise may be boring, but it's equal to an hour of running on a track, and avoids pounding and stress to the legs.

Gradually return to your regular workouts when pain has totally subsided and you have completed an adequate course of rehabilitation for two to six weeks. When you're ready to return to your former activity, massage the shins before exercise, warm up properly, and begin your workout at a greatly reduced schedule. Ice the area when you're finished to reduce any inflammation.

What the Doctor Will Do

If pain returns after you resume activity, contact your orthopedist for an examination. After taking a history, the doctor will take a bone scan and X rays to detect any minute cracks in the shin, the sign of a stress fracture. If chronic compartment syndrome is suspected in the lower leg, the doctor will take a pressure test of the sore muscle compartment with a syringe. Anti-inflammatory medication may be prescribed, or in the case of compartment syndrome, minor surgery recommended.

Prevention

Shin splints can be avoided with some common sense measures:

- Replace or repair exercise shoes that are worn down in the heels. Switch to well-fitting shoes with plenty of impact absorbing material in the forefoot and heel area. (Remember your running shoes may lose much of their shock absorbency after as few as 500 miles. Be prepared to buy a new pair.)
- Warm up before running by first walking, then gradually increase speed to a jog. When you raise your heart rate and lightly perspire, stop and stretch your calf muscles with a wall stretch.

  Wall stretch: Stand about 2 feet from a wall and place your palms flat against it. Bend your right leg slightly and stretch the left leg behind you with the knee locked straight. Keep your heel on the floor and your toes pointed straight ahead. Keeping your back straight, slowly lean toward the wall until you feel the calf of the rear leg begin to stretch. Hold this position for up to 30 seconds. Do not bounce while you stretch. Repeat with the other leg.
- Another effective way to stretch out both the tight calf muscles and Achilles tendons after warming up is to walk slowly on your heels for 100–200 yards.
- Whenever you go for a run or walk, do it on dirt, grass, cinder, or a rubberized track to minimize shin trauma.
- In an aerobics class, make sure the floor is wooden and slightly raised off the ground so it will "give" as you exercise. This will reduce impact forces.

WHAT TO DO

At the first sign of pain in the shins, stop your activity and

- Massage the area with ice to reduce inflammation and irritation.
- Take 2 ibuprofen tablets three times daily for pain relief.
- Don't apply heat to the area. This will cause increased inflammation.
- Take a break from your workouts and shift to water exercise, a bicycle, stair climber, cross-country ski machine, or other low-impact activity.
- Gradually return to regular workouts when pain has completely subsided.
- If pain returns after resuming your activity, contact your orthopedist.

SPRAINS

Joseph F. Fetto, M.D.

Dr. Fetto is associate professor of Orthopedics at the New York University Medical Center and director of the NYU Medical Center Sports Medicine Clinic in New York City

A ligament is a ropelike strand of collagen that attaches the end of one bone to another, thereby forming a joint. The ligament provides stability and support. When a joint is bent or twisted as the result of a fall, or when it's pushed beyond what the ligament can tolerate, the ligament can be stretched and torn. The tear can be microscopic, partial, or complete. The resulting stretched or torn ligament is called a sprain.

Sprains are common accidents for anyone involved in sports and fitness activities. The ankle, knee, and finger joints are particularly susceptible.

Sprains are grouped by level of severity into three categories:

Grade I sprains have only microscopic damage, resulting in minor discomfort and possible minimal swelling and discoloration. The basic structure of the ligament remains intact, and there is no permanent damage.

In Grade II sprains, the ligament is stretched and partially torn. The injury is extremely painful, accompanied by swelling and black and blue discoloration.

Grade III sprains are complete tears of the muscle or ligament and cause extensive tissue damage, discoloration, and swelling. There is little if any pain with a complete tear because when the ligament is severed, no tension occurs across the fibers that have been separated. Except for the cruciate ligaments in the knee, Grade III sprains don't always require surgery. If the ligaments remain in close contact they can possibly return to former strength provided they are allowed to heal sufficiently. *All* partially ruptured or completely severed ligaments require medical attention.

When ligaments are damaged or torn, they require a minimum of six weeks to heal completely, and up to six months for a Grade II or III injury. Although the acute injury may feel better in ten to fourteen days, don't let this lull you into a false sense of security. If you engage in intense activity too soon, you will stretch out the ligament, making it permanently lax. This can lead to a chronically unstable joint that may eventually require surgery.

Treatment

The first thing to do after you suffer a sprain is to minimize swelling with a series of actions known as RICE, an acronym for rest, ice, compression, and elevation.

Rest means to stop using the injured joint immediately to minimize stress, prevent further injury, and reduce swelling. Blood vessels start to enlarge in response to the injury and fluids flow in, causing the area to swell. This swelling leads to stiffness, can cause further disability, and slows recovery time.

Apply ice immediately to the joint to reduce inflammation. Never apply heat to a sprain because this causes blood vessels to open even wider and tissues to swell further. Ice causes the blood vessels to contract, which reduces the amount of blood around the injury.

Ice can be applied to a sprain in several ways. For injuries to the ankle, toe, wrist, or finger, fill a bucket or appropriate container with water and ice cubes and immerse the injured area in it.

For an injury to the knee, shoulder, or back use an ice pack. To prevent superficial frostbite, first put a damp towel over the skin, apply ice cubes or cracked ice that has been placed in an ice pack or sealed plastic bag. Hold the ice on the injury with your hand, or wrap it with an elastic support bandage to keep it from moving.

Keep the injured area iced for 15 minutes and then remove it for 30 minutes to allow the skin to warm up. Repeat this icing sequence for the next twenty-four to forty-eight hours.

Compression helps decrease swelling by reducing the amount of blood that can get to the area. If you have an elastic support bandage available, start by wrapping it below the injury area, directly over the ice, and then above the injured part. Don't wrap so tightly that the area becomes numb or cramped. Check your fingernails or toenails. If they appear to be blue in color, it means the wrap is too tight. Remove it, and when normal color has returned to your nails, reapply it a bit looser.

Once the initial trauma is over and swelling has stopped, the best way to keep up the compression is with an air splint. Available OTC in surgical supply stores, these lightweight, inflatable plastic casts help reduce swelling, support the area, and speed recovery by allowing you to use your joint while you rehabilitate.

Elevation of the injured body part higher than heart level greatly reduces the pooling of fluid into the damaged area. You can easily do this by lying down and propping up the injured arm or leg on pillows.

Anti-inflammatory medication such as aspirin or ibuprofen can be taken for pain relief. Aspirin will thin the blood and lead to more bleeding. Ibuprofen will also have an effect on bleeding, but not as much as aspirin. If you notice a lot of black and blue developing around the swelling, take acetaminophen for pain relief.

After twenty-four to seventy-two hours, the pain and swelling should be reduced, and you can apply heat to the injury site instead of ice. Heat from a hot shower or a bath slightly warmer than body temperature to as high as 110 degrees, a heating pad, or heat lamp are very good ways to reduce joint and ligament stiffness and help loosen the damaged tissues.

If you feel a topical liniment works for you, then apply one at this time. Gently massage it into the skin to help increase blood flow and reduce feelings of pain and stiffness. The salve may feel good on joints close to the skin such as the ankle, knee, wrist, and elbow, but for the hip and back, they prove to be less effective.

When the pain has lessened, begin to rotate the joint gingerly in all directions in an effort to restore flexibility, strength, and endurance. This will also help force some of the excess fluid out of the joint.

As a rule of thumb, for every week you're knocked out of commission due to a sprain, it takes a month to work your way safely back to your old activity level. Resume your normal activities gradually. If it is needed, continue to use an elastic support bandage or air cast for support.

Cause for Concern

Sprains can be successfully treated at home, but if there is no pain associated with a severe sprain and you have good reason to suspect a Grade III injury, or if the swelling and pain don't seem to be going away as they have in the past, contact an orthopedist for an examination to assess your injury and to rule out the possibility of a fracture.

What the Doctor Will Do

The doctor will take a history to find out how the accident happened and what mechanics were involved. A physical exam will also reveal the degree of injury. X rays and MRIs (magnetic resonance imaging) can help with further evaluation. Depending on the injury, your personality, and lifestyle, the doctor may recommend a sling, crutches, an air cast, a plaster cast, or a splint to minimize motion. Stronger prescription medication may be given for pain and inflammation relief.

WHAT TO DO

- Rest the injured body part.
- Apply ice immediately—15 minutes on, 30 minutes off—and repeat for the next twenty-four to forty-eight hours.
- Wrap the injured area and ice with an elastic bandage to reduce swelling.
- Keep the injured body part raised higher than the level of the heart to reduce swelling.
- Take acetaminophen for pain relief.
- Contact an orthopedist if you have doubts about the severity of your injury or if there is a question in your mind about the possibility of a fractured bone.

STIFF NECK

James B. Reynolds, M.D.

Dr. Reynolds is an orthopedic surgeon and staff physician at SpineCare Medical Center in Daly City, California

Neck pain can sometimes be temporarily disabling, causing headache, shoulder pain, numbness or loss of sensation in one arm, and pain that radiates from the neck and shoots to the arms and legs.

Neck pain is a common complaint after middle age. Usually it is nothing more than temporary discomfort brought on by sleeping on a soft mattress, but it can also be caused by poor posture, obesity, a muscle spasm related to exercise, or a task that requires you to bend or twist your neck. Tension and stress, which cause the muscles surrounding the neck to tense and go into spasm, can also lead to a stiff neck.

Severe neck pain can also develop from a blow to the neck, or whiplash—a violent overstretching of a muscle or ligament in the neck.

A primary cause of most neck pain is from the natural degeneration of the bones and disks of the cervical spine. The very process of aging causes the joints to wear down, producing bony spurs that press on nerves or joints that become inflamed.

The jellylike discs, which lie between the vertebrae, also begin to shrink and dry up as their water content naturally decreases with age. This degeneration may cause pain to flare up from time to time. Typical signs of degeneration include painful muscle spasms in the neck that appear suddenly and a dull aching pain in one arm.

Nerve root impingement is another source of neck pain. Following either a direct blow to the neck or degeneration of the disks, which may cause a disk to bulge or rupture, the vertebra or disk may then press or impinge on the nerves of the spine or spinal cord. Pain can be felt in the neck, shoulder, and arm, occasionally the legs.

Bone pain may also cause similar symptoms. Facet syndrome, an inflammation of the joints in the neck, is generally caused when arthritis or poor neck alignment from whiplash or a sprain of the neck ligaments causes the facets, the tiny neck joints, to swell and become painful. This may bring about excess pressure on the nerves and trigger neck or arm pain.

Luckily, the neck, more so than the lower back, responds well to conservative care and mild stretching and strengthening exercises that can be performed at home.

Treatment

Most important, when you have neck pain, is to avoid doing things that will aggravate it. Driving or riding in a car, and using a computer or typewriter are common activities that may aggravate your neck. The best way to protect your neck is to keep your head centered directly on top of your shoulders in a military posture at all times.

Don't tilt your head forward. When most people have neck pain, there is a natural tendency to let the head slump forward, but this aggravates neck pain by stretching the muscles and ligaments that surround the neck.

When you first notice your neck is stiff and sore, apply ice for upward of 20 minutes to reduce any swelling and inflammation.

An ice bag or reusable gel-pack that can be purchased in the pharmacy will work fine. My favorite form of cold treatment is a big bag of frozen peas. The peas are not intensely cold, so they won't cause frostbite of the skin. Also, they easily mold to the neck.

If you experience no relief after two days, apply a towel moistened with hot water, or an electric heating pad placed on the neck for 20 minutes three times a day. This will increase blood flow and reduce muscle soreness. In some cases it may cause extra swelling of the muscles.

Neck pain doesn't call for prolonged bed rest, but during any acute phase of neck pain, it's important to lie down flat on your back in order to take the weight off your back.

Put a rolled-up towel or a special cervical pillow from the pharmacy directly under the neck for support.

Aspirin and ibuprofen are excellent for relieving the pain and inflammation that accompany a stiff neck. I think aspirin is the better of the two but take it only if your stomach can tolerate it.

If you don't have hypersensitivity to aspirin or ulcers, or if you're not taking anticoagulant medication, take 2 aspirin every four hours. Maintaining a high level of aspirin in the blood can reduce stiffness, inflammation, and pain.

If the weather is cold outside, cover your neck with a scarf. Cold or damp air tenses the neck muscles and causes them to go into spasm.

I don't believe topical liniments help neck pain because they don't penetrate down to where the pain is located. However, liniment does act as a skin irritant and may temporarily block the transmission of pain signals, thereby diminishing pain.

Excess weight and poor posture speed up the degenerative changes in the cervical spine by tugging the cervical spine downward, placing increased pressure on the disks and vertebrae.

In order to lose weight sensibly, protect your spine, and improve overall health, make sensible food choices and begin a gradual exercise program.

Neck Stretching Exercises

Special neck stretching and strengthening exercises help restore range of motion and strength to the neck by stretching ligaments and strengthening the muscles that support your spine and head. As you perform the following exercises, you will lubricate the joints in the neck and help supply nutrition to the spinal disks.

The Exercises

Perform the following exercise during the acute and most painful stage of your neck pain:

- *Head retraction.* While sitting, relax and look straight ahead. Keep your chin tucked down and *slowly* move your head backward as far as you can while continuing to look forward. To achieve further extension, place your fingers on your chin and gently push back.

  Do not look up. When the head is back as far as you can possibly move it, hold the position for a few seconds, then relax and return to the starting position. Repeat ten times and perform the exercise six to eight times throughout the course of the day.

  When the acute phase has *subsided,* perform the following exercise:

- *Neck extension.* After performing the head retraction exercise, immediately

follow with this exercise. With your head retracted back to the farthest position, tilt your chin up and look straight up to the ceiling.

Move your nose a half inch to the right of center, hold for the count of 3, return to the midline, and then tilt your nose to the left a half-inch and hold for the count of 3. As you tilt your nose, try to move the neck and head back even farther. Repeat this right-left cycle ten times and then perform the exercise six to eight times during the course of the day.

- *Chin on chest.* While sitting, flex your neck slowly forward and try to touch your chin to your chest. Hold the stretch at your chest for 10 seconds and return to the starting position. Repeat five times.

- *Head on shoulders.* While sitting, slowly tilt your head straight back and try to touch your upper head to your shoulders. Hold the stretch for 10 seconds and return to the starting position. Repeat five times.

- *Side head bends.* While sitting, look straight ahead and slowly tilt your head to the right and try to touch your right ear to your right shoulder. This gently stretches the left side of the neck. Don't raise your shoulder to meet your head. Hold the stretch for 10 seconds and return to the starting position. Repeat five times, and then perform the stretch on the left side.

Neck Strengthening Exercises

Isometric exercises, in which you contract your neck muscles and push against a fixed resistance, help to decrease swelling of the neck muscles and also provide gains in overall strength.

- *Forehead push.* While sitting, place palms of both hands on the forehead. Tense the neck muscles and try to push forward. Resist with the palms so the head can't move. Hold this position for 10 seconds and repeat five times.
- *Head push-up.* Tilt the head slightly forward, interlace your fingers, and place your palms on the back of the head. Try to push up against the resistance of the palms without moving your head. Hold for 10 seconds and repeat five times.
- *Side head bend.* Place your right hand to the side of your head and try to move your head to your right shoulder while providing resistance with your hand. Do not let the head move. Hold the position for 10 seconds, repeat five times, and then perform the same exercise on the left side.

Cause for Concern

Contact a doctor immediately if you simultaneously twist your neck and shoulder in opposite directions while playing any contact sport and feel a burning sensation in your neck. This neck pain, commonly called a cervical "burner," occurs after aggressively stretching the shoulder and neck, which in turn stretches the cervical nerves that branch off the spinal cord to the neck. This results in shooting, burning pain, and often will lead to muscle weakness and loss of sensation in the shoulder area.

Also, contact a doctor immediately if you have a stiff neck accompanied by vomiting and extreme lethargy. These are three signs of meningitis, a viral or bacterial inflammation of the covering of the brain and spinal column. It requires immediate treatment.

What the Doctor Will Do

There is no need to call a doctor immediately for simple neck pain or aches. However, if after a week of self-care the pain seems to be the same or is getting worse, contact your family doctor.

The doctor will take a history to find out the source of the injury, perform a physical exam to check the muscles and tendons of the neck for signs of tenderness or spasm, and test the flexion of your neck by having you gently move your neck in all directions. He will also check the strength and reflexes of your arms and legs. He may also wish to take an X ray at this time.

In most cases, physical therapy is prescribed. Cervical collars, the soft devices worn around the neck to prevent movement, generally tend to weaken the neck muscles and aren't typically prescribed unless there is severe pain or damage.

WHAT TO DO

- Avoid doing things during the course of the day that will aggravate the neck.
- Keep your head centered at all times directly on top of your shoulders in a military posture.
- Don't tilt your head forward.
- Apply ice to your neck for upward of 20 minutes when you first notice your neck is stiff, sore, or painful.

- If no relief is obtained with ice two days after the onset of neck pain, apply heat.
- Lie down on your back during an acute phase of neck pain.
- Avoid using a pillow that flexes or tilts the neck upward.
- Place a rolled-up towel, a small pillow, or a cervical pillow under the neck to fill the gap between the head and shoulders.
- Take 2 aspirin every four hours if your stomach can tolerate it.
- Cover your neck with a scarf if the weather is cold outside.
- If extremely overweight, lose weight through regular exercise and proper food choices.
- Perform special neck stretching and strengthening exercises to restore range of motion and strength to the neck.
- Contact your physician immediately if you have a stiff neck that is accompanied by vomiting and extreme lethargy. These are symptoms of meningitis.
- If the neck pain seems to be the same, or is getting worse after one week of self-care, contact your doctor for an examination.

TENDINITIS

Charles B. Goodwin, M.D.

Dr. Goodwin is clinical instructor in Orthopedic Surgery at Columbia/Presbyterian Medical Center in New York City, attending orthopedic surgeon at St. Luke's/Roosevelt Hospital Center, New York City and orthopedic consultant to the U.S. Open Tennis Tournament

Whenever you ask your body to go beyond the ordinary range of motion; or perform an activity that requires great force to push, pull, or lift; or repeatedly flex a joint such as a wrist, knee, or elbow, your tendons can become stressed and irritated. The pain, stiffness, and swelling that develops is known as tendinitis.

A tendon is a fibrous, ropelike strand of tissue that crosses a joint, connecting muscle to bone. When stressed, tendons develop microscopic tears and become painfully inflamed. Tendinitis is most common in the forty-to-fifty age bracket, among people who are still fairly athletic. But when their minds say *yes,* their bodies too often answer *maybe.*

Tendinitis typically develops when a person goes directly to the tennis court, for example, and instead of warming up his serve gradually, yells out, "First one in" and starts hitting the ball as hard as possible. Or it can begin when a person goes to the first tee or practice area to hit a bucket of balls, swinging full force with the driver before doing stretching exercises.

Tendinitis can also develop at an earlier age if you're a competitive athlete who trains daily, or if you're a regular exerciser who performs the same workout day after day. It can also develop if your job requires the same repetitive movement during the work day.

Tendinitis is most painful when you wake up in the morning. Once you move around, the body warms up and the inflammation diminishes. However, it comes back as strong as ever once the body cools down again.

Treatment

Tendinitis can be treated, but only when the cause is identified and allowed time for healing. Depending on the degree of inflammation, tendinitis usually disappears in a few days, but can linger for weeks in more severe cases.

If you've developed tendinitis, you need ice, some anti-inflammatory medication, and rest. Ice should be applied at the *initial* sign of tendon pain, and this means even a barely recognizable soreness or dull ache. Ice helps quell the inflammation and reduce any swelling.

The best way I've found to ice an inflamed joint is to fill a plastic bag with ice and a little water. The water helps the cold diffuse more quickly. Knot the open end of the bag with a rubber band to seal it off. Place the ice directly on the joint and leave it there for 20 minutes.

For relief from inflammation, take 2 aspirin or ibuprofen tablets, four to six times a day depending on the severity of the symptoms. The most common side effect of this medication is stomach irritation. Anti-inflammatory medication is contraindicated if you have peptic ulcer disease. Check with your physician first. Acetaminophen is a pain medication and doesn't decrease the inflammation of tendinitis.

A good preventive measure is to take your medication *before* you perform your work or sport. This way, the drug will keep the tendon from flaring up as you exercise or work.

Rest is important to stop further inflammation and give the tendon a chance to heal. Don't resume your activity at full tilt until the pain has completely gone away or you risk aggravating the injury.

Apply an elastic support bandage to the sore area. This reduces swelling through gentle compression and serves as a reminder to take it easy. To immobilize the arm or shoulder and prevent further damage, wear a sling.

After twenty-four to forty-eight hours, depending on the degree of pain, apply heat to the area to increase blood flow and speed up the removal of inflammatory byproducts. This can be done with a hot shower or bath, or a heating pad. Liniments can be beneficial at this time because the hot, tingling sensation they bring to the area helps block the pain signals sent to the brain.

Once the pain has diminished, rehabilitation begins. Whether you're an athlete or nonathlete, if your muscles aren't properly conditioned they will not adequately support your joints, and you're liable to reinjure yourself. Specific exercises should be started to get back the range of motion to the joint and increase muscular strength. If you don't do any exercises, the joint will get stiff and prolong your recovery.

Here is a way to restore flexion to the knee. Sit in a chair with your feet flat on the floor in front of you. Slowly bring your heel back to the front of the chair.

To strengthen your injured knee, sit on the floor with your leg out in front of you. Push down on your extended leg and flex your quadricep muscles, the muscle group on the top of the thigh. Hold the flex for the count of 6 and then relax. Repeat five times.

To get back range of motion in an injured shoulder, try gentle pendulum exercises. While standing with your knees locked, bend over slowly at the waist as far as you can so your chest is parallel to the floor. Let your arm hang down like a pendulum and then gently swing it in a circle. Also, pretend that you have a bowling ball in your hand and gently swing the arm backward and forward as if you were bowling. Continue for 2 minutes, and repeat the drill every twelve hours.

Tennis elbow occurs when you excessively or improperly contract the muscles of your forearm. This strains the tendons that connect the muscles to the elbow. This common form of tendinitis is not limited to racket sports, but can develop from gardening, lifting luggage, and even shaking hands.

The best defense is to build up strength in the forearm muscles. When pain diminishes, several times throughout the day squeeze a hand grip, a tennis ball, or a wadded-up ball of paper on and off for 2 minutes, or until the forearm fatigues.

Another effective exercise is to grasp a 3-pound hand weight and hang your wrist over the end of a table with your palm down. Gently extend your wrist outward and then return to the starting point. Repeat fifteen times.

What the Doctor Will Do

If these conservative measures fail to bring relief, contact your orthopedist. Depending on the severity of your tendinitis, the doctor may prescribe stronger anti-inflammatory medication or recommend prednisone, a corticosteroid taken for eight to ten days. In addition, a physical therapy session may be prescribed.

WHAT TO DO

- Rest. Stop the activity that directly causes the pain.
- Apply ice to the painful area at the first sign of pain to reduce inflammation and swelling.
- Take 2 aspirin or ibuprofen tablets four to six times daily if you can tolerate it.
- Use an elastic support wrap or sling to compress and immobilize the affected body part.
- Apply heat twenty-four to forty-eight hours after pain symptoms have diminished to speed up the healing process.
- Perform appropriate muscle stretching and then strengthening exercises when soreness has decreased.
- Contact your orthopedist if you still have pain after several days of self-treatment.

Teeth and Mouth

GENERAL INFORMATION

Besides cutting and grinding food, teeth help maintain facial contour and form the spoken word. Most adults have thirty-two permanent teeth: twelve molars, eight premolars, four canines, and eight incisors.

Enamel, the hardest substance in the body, covers the outside of the tooth. Tooth enamel can be broken down by plaque, a combination of bacteria, sugar, and saliva that forms a film on teeth. Plaque can produce acids and enzymes strong enough to erode tooth enamel and form a fissure or crack, which in turn may lead to decay.

Dentin, a substance similar to bone but denser, is located just inside the enamel. It comprises the largest part of the tooth and is made up of millions of cells. Just inside the dentin is the pulp, where blood vessels and nerves supply the cells that form the dentin. The jawbone and gum (gingiva) surround and support the teeth.

Tooth decay, gum disease, and the chance of tooth loss can be minimized for most people with oral hygiene, brushing at least twice daily and using dental floss once a day. Two dental checkups each year for examination and tooth cleaning complete these procedures.

DENTAL SPECIALISTS

GENERAL DENTIST (D.D.S. or D.M.D.). A dentist is a physician concerned with the diagnosis and treatment of diseases of the teeth, jaw, and gums.

ENDODONTIST. A dentist who diagnoses and treats diseases of the tooth pulp, usually by performing root canal work.

ORAL AND MAXILLOFACIAL SURGEON. Performs extractions and treats diseases and injuries to the mouth, jaw, and face.

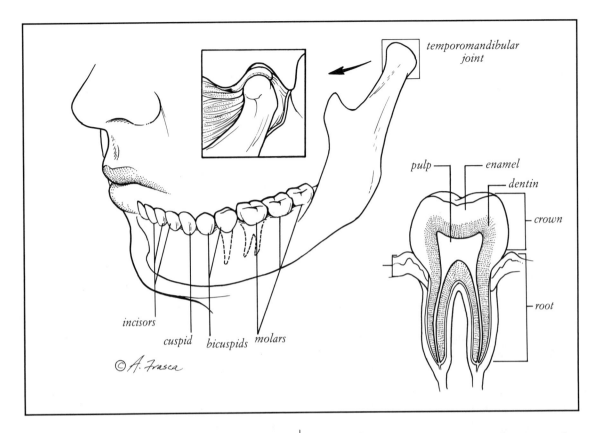

temporomandibular joint

pulp — *enamel*
dentin
crown
root

incisors
cuspid *bicuspids* *molars*

© A. Frasca

ORAL PATHOLOGIST. A dentist who diagnoses and treats medical problems of the oral mucosa (mucus membrane, lining of the mouth) and jaws through clinical and microscopic evaluation (biopsy).

ORTHODONTIST. Treats malocclusion of the teeth (misalignment) with dental appliances (braces). The orthodontist sometimes works in conjunction with an oral surgeon if extraction or surgery are advised.

PEDODONTIST. This pediatric dentist specializes in the dental care of children.

PERIODONTIST. A dentist who treats diseases of the tissue supporting the teeth, chiefly the jawbone and gums, and restores lost teeth with the use of dental implants.

PROSTHODONTIST. A specialist who designs and fits dentures, bridges, and caps.

DENTAL EMERGENCY

BROKEN TOOTH. When a tooth is knocked out or fragmented by a blow, find the fragments of the tooth and put into a liquid or wrap in a moist cloth. Get to a doctor or hospital Emergency Department as quickly as possible. Optimum time to *continued on page 100*

COMMON MOUTH AND TEETH PROBLEMS

BAD BREATH
A temporary or chronic problem, stemming from poor dental hygiene, trapped food particles, poorly fitting crowns or dentures, tooth decay, pungent foods, or from problems relating to the lung, nose, throat, or stomach. It can also be a symptom of systemic disease such as diabetes.

Page 100

CANKER SORES
A small painful mouth ulcer—round, symmetrical, slightly raised, and with a red halo border. Typically found on the inside of the cheek, soft palate, inner lip, or side of the tongue.

Page 103

TEETH GRINDING
Bruxism, the grinding of the upper and lower teeth while sleeping; it usually requires no medical treatment.

Page 105

TEETHING
A normal, sometimes painful, process in which the twenty primary teeth come into the mouth. Teething usually begins at six months and continues through age three. Permanent tooth eruption, especially of the wisdom teeth, may also be accompanied by discomfort.

Page 106

TMJ
This often overdiagnosed jaw ailment is typified by chronic jaw pain and difficulty in opening the mouth and chewing.

Page 107

TOOTHACHE
Pain of varying intensity develops in the tooth due to decay or trauma.

Page 109

repair a damaged tooth is within two hours of the accident.

DENTIST'S CARE REQUIRED

GUM DISEASE. Also called periodontitis or pyorrhea. This gum infection is the leading cause of tooth loss among adults. Symptoms include bad breath, bleeding gums, and, in advanced stages, loosened teeth.

IMPACTED TOOTH. When the third molar (the wisdom tooth) begins to grow in, it is often too large for the jaw. This forces the new tooth to press against the adjacent molar, and it becomes impacted (blocked). Intense pain and infection may result. The tooth is often extracted.

TOOTH ABSCESS. Pus-filled sac that forms around the root of a tooth, caused by decay or receding gums. Throbbing pain, extreme sensitivity to hot and cold liquids, and swollen neck glands are common symptoms. An abscess can be treated with a thorough cleaning and filling, or extraction.

TRENCH MOUTH. Painful bacterial infection of the gums, typically in the area between the teeth. Relatively rare, it is caused by poor oral hygiene and nutrition, throat infection, or smoking. Trench mouth is also known as ulcerative gingivitis or Vincent's infection. Principal symptom is red, swollen, painful gums that bleed easily.

BAD BREATH

Michael K. Sonick, D.M.D.

Dr. Sonick is an assistant clinical professor of Periodontics at the University of Connecticut School of Dental Medicine and an active member of the teaching staff at Yale–New Haven Hospital

Bad breath, or halitosis, is caused primarily by gingivitis, a disease that develops when bacterial plaque builds up at the gum margin and between the teeth.

Plaque is a mixture of saliva, bacteria, and carbohydrates that forms daily on the teeth surface. If not removed, it results in minor infection of the gums and bad breath.

Bad breath may also occur when food is trapped between the teeth and begins to be broken down by the hundreds of bacteria that live in the mouth. Food can easily become lodged in poorly fitting dental work, broken fillings or fillings that are too large for the teeth, and in crowns that don't fit properly.

Bad breath can also arise from the tongue. The tongue has tiny hairlike projections called filiform papillae, which trap food and debris. Certain sulfur-containing medications and even some mouthwashes can get into these projections and cause bad odors. Tobacco tars from cigarettes can also leave a foul-smelling brown coating on the tongue. To eliminate this mouth odor, one must stop smoking, then brush the *tongue* twice daily for a week to remove the residue of tar and nicotine.

If you are unable to stop smoking or have to remain on the sulfur-containing medications, you must incorporate a daily brushing of the tongue as part of a program of oral hygiene to keep the mouth odor under control.

Bad breath can also be caused by disorders that don't occur in the mouth. Problems in the lungs, throat, and nose such as pneumonia, tonsillitis, or sinusitis can also cause bad breath. Stomach ailments, including heartburn (gastroesophageal reflux), are also offenders. Uncontrolled diabetics can also have bad breath due to ketoacidosis, an insulin deficiency in which body fats are burned in the absence of sufficient body sugars. This same reaction will cause bad breath by the second day of a food fast. The burning of body fats release acids that can cause bad breath.

Treatment

Halitosis-causing plaque that forms on the teeth above the gums can be brushed off with a soft-bristled toothbrush. Normal brushing can also remove the plaque 2–3 mm below the gums. Flossing once a day will get rid of plaque that tends to form between the teeth. But even if you brush and floss well, you can't reach the plaque that forms deep below the gum line, and this plaque could be responsible for chronic bad breath.

Mouthwashes contain chemicals and oils that are useful in killing bacteria in the mouth. These rinses work well on bacteria that is above the gumline and may have some effect in combating gum inflammation, but they are not effective in treating periodontal disease because they can't get into the pockets between the teeth.

Thus, although mouthwashes help reduce the amount of plaque in the mouth, removing plaque is better done with a toothbrush and floss. However, if you like to use mouthwash to feel fresher after brushing and flossing, that's fine.

Mints and breath candies formulated to combat bad breath actually just mask it by introducing a mentholated or mint odor. For bad breath brought on by certain foods, these mints can help temporarily. However, bad breath will return in anywhere from a few minutes to an hour. If the breath mint has sugar in it, it will only exacerbate the problem by feeding the bacteria in your mouth and causing them to increase.

If you are dining out and don't have access to a toothbrush, take a mouthful of water, swish it around, and either swallow or spit it out. This will help to alleviate the problem of bad breath temporarily.

Dentures—removable artificial teeth that fit over the gum in the absence of natural teeth—are also a primary source of bad breath, a bad taste in the mouth, and infection if they don't fit properly.

To prevent bad breath stemming from dentures, contact your dentist if you notice any space between the denture and the gum. This is a major site for plaque buildup. Brush and clean dentures daily, and take them out at night to let the gum tissues "breathe." To prevent infection in the soft tissue of the mouth, rinse the mouth well to keep the gums clean.

Cause for Concern

Chronic bad breath may be caused by a gum infection called gingivitis. Typical early symptoms include swollen and red gums that bleed easily when the teeth are brushed.

Gingivitis has to be treated by a dentist or it may advance to a more serious condition called periodontitis. Periodontitis can cause loss of gum tissue and bone, and the breakdown of the supporting structure of the teeth. If uncorrected, teeth may eventually loosen and fall out.

Most people with gingivitis don't realize they have bad breath. A simple way to find out is to cup your hands in front of your face, gently blow into them, and quickly inhale. If your breath smells bad to you, it probably will smell bad to others as well. But even if this test seems to come up negative, you may still have bad breath.

A second self-test is more definitive. Take a piece of dental floss and floss between your back molars, using a gentle back and forth sawing motion going down to the gum line. Smell that area of the floss when you're done. If it smells bad, it's a good bet that you have bad breath and possibly gingivitis.

If bad breath becomes long-standing, contact your dentist. However, if you and your dentist can't link it with any dental cause, or if you think it may be related to some serious condition, contact your physician.

Prevention

- Brush teeth daily with a soft-bristled brush and fluoridated toothpaste.
- Floss teeth once a day.
- Have teeth examined and cleaned twice a year by a dentist.

WHAT TO DO

- Brush the teeth twice daily with a soft brush and floss once a day.
- Scrub the tongue with a toothbrush to remove the brown or black film of bacteria, cigarette tars, and food debris.
- Stop smoking.
- Use a mouthwash to kill some plaque-forming bacteria and freshen the mouth temporarily.
- Be wary of breath mints. They will mask mouth odor temporarily, but could heighten odor later because the sugar in the mint nourishes mouth bacteria.
- If you don't have access to a toothbrush, swish water around in your mouth, and either swallow or spit it out.

To prevent bad breath stemming from denture wear:
- Make sure dentures fit properly.
- Brush and clean dentures daily.
- Take dentures out at night to let the gums "breathe."
- Rinse the mouth well to keep the gums clean.
- If you and your dentist can't link bad breath with any dental cause, or if you think it may be related to a lung, nose, or gastrointestinal problem, contact your physician.

CANKER SORES

Ellen Eisenberg, D.M.D.

Dr. Eisenberg is associate professor of Oral Diagnosis, Division of Oral Pathology, at the University of Connecticut School of Dental Medicine in Farmington, Connecticut

A canker sore, medically known as a recurrent aphthous ulcer, is a fairly common mouth lesion that affects between 20 and 60 percent of the adolescent to fifty-year-old population. A canker sore usually heals itself in fourteen days and may recur several times a year, but some unfortunate people are almost never without them.

These ulcers are usually found on the inside of the cheek. They are slightly raised above the oral surface, round in shape, and typically have a white or yellow center with a red halo around the border. They vary in size from several millimeters to greater than a centimeter.

They may appear alone or in a cluster in the area at the base of the gums, the inner lip, on the tongue, or on the soft palate at the back of the mouth. Even though they are small, canker sores are intensely painful.

Canker sores are not related to viruses, but may be caused by a variety of factors all working in concert with your own immune system. Stress and emotional tension seem to be some of the conditions that trigger canker sores. Women may find that canker sores appear just before menstruation.

Food doesn't cause canker sores directly but can certainly aggravate them. Foods rich in citric acid (such as oranges, lemons, or tomatoes) will cause the sores to sting, as will spicy foods or food containing vinegar. Biting yourself accidentally or rubbing your toothbrush across a sore may trigger a canker sore but does not directly cause one to develop.

Treatment

There is no cure for canker sores, but the pain from them can be eased with some home remedies and products prescribed by your dentist.

Apply crushed ice to the lesion. This will numb the pain and provide some temporary relief.

Before meals, a mixture of 1 tablespoonful of bismuth salicylate (Kaopectate) with equal parts lidocaine and diphenhydramine elixir (Benadryl) may be helpful. The pharmacist will make it up for you on the dentist's prescription. Swish this mixture around the mouth for a couple of minutes to provide good coating of the sores, and then spit it out. It may offer a protective barrier against the foods you plan to eat.

Cause for Concern

If home remedies don't help, or if your canker sore hasn't gotten better after two weeks, or if you suffer from recurring bouts, it is advisable to contact your dentist. Canker sores make up a large percentage of the chronic oral ulcers or sores a dentist can diagnose and manage.

What the Doctor Will Do

For people who keep getting canker sores, a variety of different medical treatments can be prescribed by your dentist to relieve pain and speed healing. For prompt relief, the oral antibiotic tetracycline may help. This is swished around in the mouth for several minutes at a time, three times daily. In lieu of this, gauze may be soaked in the tetracycline solution and placed against the lesion for as long as it can be tolerated.

The dentist may also prescribe a topical steroid ointment or swish. In severe cases, corticosteroids in tablet form may be prescribed. This medicine cuts recovery time considerably. For frequently recurring cases, corticosteroid medication may be prescribed prophylactically (preventively) for a period of several weeks to lessen the frequency and severity of future bouts.

Dentists can take an aggressive, short-term drug approach to canker sores when someone is plagued by them. This requires thorough familiarity with available drugs and knowledge of how to prescribe them wisely. If you can find an oral pathologist or oral medicine specialist, he or she would be the one most familiar with effective management of recurrent canker sores.

WHAT TO DO

- Avoid aggravating the canker sore. Don't eat spicy foods or foods rich in citric acid or vinegar while the lesions are present.
- Avoid physically injuring the affected tissue through cheek biting or eating hard, abrasive foods.
- Be careful not to injure the tissue with a toothbrush or utensil.
- Apply crushed ice to the sore to numb the pain.
- For a temporary protective coating, the pharmacist can make a prescribed mixture of bismuth salicylate (Kaopectate), lidocaine, and diphenhydramine elixir (Benadryl), which can be used before meals. Swish it around the mouth for a minute or two and spit out.
- If these measures don't work and your canker sore hasn't gotten better in two weeks, or if you suffer from chronic canker sores, contact your dentist or oral pathologist. Prescribed short-term topical or systemic steroid therapy may help relieve the pain and speed recovery during each outbreak. It may also diminish frequency of occurrence.

TEETH GRINDING

Joseph J. Marbach, D.D.S.

*Dr. Marbach is clinical professor of public health (sociomedical science), at the
School of Public Health, at Columbia University in New York City*

Bruxism is the habit of grinding the teeth together, typically at night.

Although the grating noise may be annoying for a spouse or sibling, teeth grinding is not something to become worried about.

Contrary to popular belief, chronic teeth grinding will rarely wear down your teeth, nor does bruxism have a link with temporomandibular joint syndrome (see TMJ, page 107). And there is little that can be done to stop bruxism, which is thought to be transmitted genetically and occurs in 20 percent of all people.

There is some evidence that emotional or physical stress can lead to nocturnal teeth grinding, which may be a way to relieve tension. People who exhibit temporary bruxism also toss and turn in their sleep, perspire heavily, and exhibit other symptoms typical of stress that are not related specifically to bruxism. All of my studies indicate that once these people solve their problems, their symptoms, including teeth grinding, vanish.

Treatment

I don't recommend bite plates and see no reason for them. There is no evidence that they prevent teeth grinding, and if a dentist recommends one, question the reasons for it. Two groups of people habitually grind their teeth: those who have a family link with teeth grinding and people who get bite plates from dentists. These bite plates are made of plastic or rubber and are also known as tooth guards or splints. So if a dentist gives you a bite plate, you will likely end up chewing on it as well.

Cause for Concern

There are two things to remember about teeth grinding. The teeth are the hardest structures in the body and the chance of wearing them down by grinding, except in very rare instances when there are other disorders involved, is extremely remote. However, if you notice any signs of worn enamel, contact your dentist. Filler material may have to replace the lost enamel.

WHAT TO DO

- Seek counseling or psychotherapy, or try stress-reduction exercises.
- Contact your dentist if you notice any abnormal enamel erosion. It could be a sign of an underlying dental disorder.

TEETHING

Heber Simmons, Jr., D.D.S.

Dr. Simmons is the past president of the American Academy of Pediatric Dentistry
and a pediatric dentist in Jackson, Mississippi

The process of growing twenty baby teeth is called teething. These teeth usually arrive at six months of age and continue arriving two at a time on a regular basis until the child is three years old.

Teething is often a painful experience for a child, because the teeth have to push through the gum pad to emerge. Symptoms include red and swollen gum pads, drooling, crankiness, and sleep disturbance. Teething is a natural process, and these painful symptoms can be treated effectively at home.

Treatment

Many people relieve the distress of teething with rubber teething rings. They do work sometimes, but I've rarely been able to get a child to chew on one. There are OTC preparations formulated for teething pain, but they taste terrible, and I don't think they work well at numbing the pain. Therefore, I recommend a way to ease teething pain by cleaning the baby's gums, starting as soon as mother and child get home from the hospital. Babies come to like the gentle pressure on the gums, and when the teeth begin to emerge and feel uncomfortable, this pressure is quite soothing to them.

To clean the gums, take a piece of gauze, wrap it around your forefinger and just rub it gently on the baby's gum pads. When the teeth start coming in, keep up your cleaning. This gets the bacteria off the gums and breaks up the bacterial pockets that tend to form when the teeth push through. By eliminating bacteria, you cut down on infections that lead to pain.

Once the tooth has fully emerged, clean it with fluoride toothpaste. At first it's easier to apply a small bit onto the gauze pad and rub it on the tooth with your finger. Fluoride helps hold down cavities, and your elbow grease cleans the tooth. Be sure to remove all excess paste from the baby's mouth when you're done.

Pain, drooling, and discomfort are the major symptoms associated with teething. Flushed red cheeks, loss of appetite, disturbed sleep, and a tendency to put fingers in the mouth are also common. Many other problems—from earache to sinus distress to fever—are mistakenly linked with teething, but these are *not* associated with the emergence of teeth. Anytime your baby runs a fever 1 degree above normal, consult your pediatrician.

Cause for Concern

As first-year molars (the broad teeth used for grinding) emerge in the back of the mouth, a child literally has to chew the painful tissue that is now covering the new teeth. Trimming back the flap of bright red skin that surrounds a partially erupted molar does not help, and it should not be done. Leave the skin alone, and let it shrink away naturally.

WHAT TO DO

- Gently wipe the baby's gum pads daily throughout infancy with a piece of gauze wrapped around your forefinger.
- Use a small drop of fluoridated toothpaste applied to a piece of gauze to clean newly emerged teeth.
- Don't cut or remove the flap of red or inflamed skin covering newly emerging teeth. This may lead to infection.
- High fever is rare with teething. Consult with your pediatrician whenever your child runs a temperature 1 degree above normal.

TMJ

John E. Dodes, D.D.S.

Dr. Dodes is president of the National Council Against Health Fraud, New York Chapter, and is a dentist in private practice in Woodhaven, New York

Clinically diagnosed TMJ, or temporomandibular joint syndrome, is a disorder of unknown origin that primarily causes the facial muscles involved in chewing to go into spasm.

The temporomandibular joint (from "tempora," the temples, and "mandible," the lower jaw) is located in front of the ear and attaches the lower jaw to the skull. However, this joint rarely has anything to do with the problem. Nor does TMJ have anything to do with the way your upper and lower teeth fit together in your mouth.

Although researchers aren't sure, TMJ disorders may stem from a muscle problem that can affect either side of the face. The major symptom is chronic, often excruciating facial pain. This is almost always accompanied by difficulty in opening the mouth wide. The clicking or grinding noise you may hear when you open your mouth or chew is normal and doesn't signal TMJ problems as many people believe. If your jaw makes popping noises when you chew,

it's nothing to worry about. It's just the way your jaw happens to work.

A simple rule of thumb that quickly dismisses the possibility of having TMJ: If you don't have chronic facial pain, you don't have TMJ.

Treatment

The good news about TMJ is that it is self-limiting, and we have *effective* ways to treat the symptoms to speed up the healing process.

For almost 90 percent of people with TMJ, relief comes with little or no treatment at all. However, you can feel relief faster if you use some basic home treatments. (If you are not helped by these remedies, seek professional help from a neurologist, not a dentist.)

I'm sure my own TMJ is brought on by clenching and grinding my teeth in my sleep (see TEETH GRINDING, page 105). Sometimes when I wake up after a night of clenching, I feel pain and soreness between my mouth and ear.

When confronted with TMJ pain, I rely on several simple, safe, and effective remedies. First, I take 2 ibuprofen tablets for pain relief. I then apply a warm, moist washcloth to my jaw for a few minutes. When the cloth cools, I warm it again and repeat the procedure. This moist heat has a soothing effect on the jaw muscles and helps take them out of spasm.

I follow this up with a series of jaw-stretching exercises. Unlike other muscles of the body, the facial muscles are difficult to relax when they go into spasm, because they're used twice a minute, twenty-four hours a day in swallowing. However, these exercises help greatly.

For the first exercise, make a fist and place it under your chin. Press lightly into the chin and then slowly open your mouth against the pressure. Hold for the count of 3. Close your mouth. Repeat ten times.

For the next exercise, open your mouth as wide as possible without pain and then close. Repeat ten times.

Repeat both stretching drills four times daily for two days. The pain should soon clear up, and if you're lucky, stay away for four to five months. As soon as you feel the first hint of TMJ returning, start the stretching exercises once again.

TMJ symptoms will also be relieved by switching to a soft diet until the pain goes away. This means eating cereals, soups, and pastas and avoiding steak and any other hard-to-chew foods. By all means, avoid chewing gum. Excessive chewing will only serve to exacerbate or prolong the problem.

Cause for Concern

If you don't see improvement from this conservative therapy within three or four weeks, you should seek medical help from a neurologist, or go to a special TMJ clinic staffed by neurologists, physicians, dentists, and psychologists. Conservative therapies that do not require a permanent change in your teeth or jaw should be used to relieve your symptoms.

By all means, avoid dentists who want to treat TMJ by performing procedures that will change the way your teeth come together. In particular, don't let a dentist fit you with a plastic device called a MORA (mandibular orthopedic repositioning appliance). You will be told to wear this overpriced gadget all day and all night, and it may go on for years. MORAs haven't proved to be effective in treating TMJ and often destroy the alignment of the teeth.

TMJ is an ailment that is often misdiagnosed by dentists. Many of them are unscrupulous or uninformed doctors who perform needless root canal work, incorrectly recommend braces or crowns, use orthodontic appliances inappropriately, grind down teeth, and initiate invasive oral surgery, which sometimes includes breaking the jaw and inserting artificial joint replacements, as ways to "treat" this ailment. Be willing to question your dentist about the appropriateness of a recommended treatment.

WHAT TO DO

- Take 2 aspirin, acetaminophen, or ibuprofen tablets every four hours.
- Use a warm, moist compress on the affected area.

- Perform jaw-stretching exercises, ten repetitions, four times daily.
- Switch to a soft food diet.
- Don't chew gum.

- If these conservative remedies fail to bring relief, contact a neurologist or go to a TMJ clinic staffed with a neurologist, dentist, and psychologist.

TOOTHACHE

Christine Dumas, D.D.S.

Dr. Dumas is an assistant clinical professor of dentistry at the University of Southern California Dental School in Los Angeles

Toothaches are most often caused by cavities and infections and can vary in severity from a dull ache to unremitting throbbing. When you have a toothache, a dentist has to be contacted as soon as possible. But when the pain comes on in the middle of the night or you are on vacation, far from your dentist, treating yourself can offer temporary relief.

Treatment

The origin of a toothache can be as simple as a kernel of popcorn trapped between your teeth or as complex as a cracked or abscessed tooth. However, your first concern when you have a toothache is finding a way to alleviate the pain and discomfort as quickly as possible.

To take the edge off of a toothache and related gum pain before going to the dentist, take 2 ibuprofen or aspirin tablets every four hours. Two acetaminophen tablets can be substituted if you have difficulty with either aspirin or ibuprofen. These pain relievers can help minimize the discomfort, but if the pain is very sharp and the medication doesn't make it subside, the tooth's nerve is probably exposed.

If the toothache is a child's, do not give any pain or fever medication until you've contacted the dentist or pediatrician.

Never put anything directly on the tooth to relieve pain. Many people think if aspirin works so well when swallowed, it will work even better if it's crushed and applied directly to the tooth. This is the worst thing you can do. Aspirin can burn the gum tissue and cause it to slough off, and in extreme cases can lead to permanent nerve damage.

If toothache is caused by trapped food, use dental floss to clear the particles from the affected area. Guide the floss through, careful to avoid cutting the gums. If you can't remove the object, leave it alone until you see your dentist. Don't try to remove the object with a sharp or pointed instrument because you will cause more damage.

Often, with this type of dental ailment, the gums and the surrounding structures are the cause of the problem, not the tooth itself. With gingival (gum) inflammation, the teeth will usually be sensitive to biting pressure. This is frequently a low-grade ache, rather than the sharper, throbbing pain most commonly associated with a toothache.

You can rinse your mouth with tepid salted water to help relieve toothache pain. To make a salt-water rinse, add 1 teaspoon of table salt to an 8-ounce glass of warm water. Swish it around your mouth in the area of infection and spit it out. Do not use cold or hot water for this rinsing, because extremes of temperature will increase the pain. If the toothache is due to a lost filling and the nerve isn't exposed (you can tell by the level of discomfort when rinsing), you can cover the space temporarily by using a nonprescription dental powder available from your local drugstore that mixes with water to form a temporary filling paste.

An effective home remedy for pain is oil of cloves. Moisten a small cotton ball with the oil of this nonprescription product and dab it on the affected tooth with tweezers. Clove oil acts as a natural painkiller.

A toothache caused by an infection often involves swelling around the gum. After calling the dentist, the first thing I would do is go to the refrigerator and get ice cubes—or a cold can of soda if I were away from home—and place it on the cheek of the affected side for at least 15 minutes of each hour. The cold draws fluids away from the tooth and gum, relieving pressure and thereby reducing pain.

Avoid exercise when you have a toothache. Any energetic movement that gets your heart pumping and causes you to breathe in huge amounts of air over the tooth will make it throb even more.

I recommend that you reconsider flying when you have a toothache, no matter how minor you think the pain. What you may judge to be slight tooth discomfort at sea level could easily turn into agony at 30,000 feet. Similar pressure-related problems will occur if you go scuba diving when you have a toothache. The change in pressure can affect problem teeth by causing the fluid inside them to expand and press against the nerve, turning minor discomfort into excruciating pain.

Prevention

Toothache caused by decay is most effectively prevented by brushing after every meal with fluoridated toothpaste, flossing between the teeth, and seeing your dentist regularly. Your dentist can help by catching problems in their early stages before they escalate into major difficulties.

Protect teeth from trauma while playing contact sports by wearing tooth guards and other forms of protective gear. Tooth guards are available in sporting goods stores, or your dentist can make one for you.

What the Dentist Will Do

If your dentist finds infection of the tooth on examination, some minor decay removal will be carried out on that visit and a temporary filling will generally seal the tooth and protect it from food particles. The dentist won't finish his work during this initial visit because the treatment is often complex.

In cases of suspected infection, antibiotics are often prescribed for several days. Because infection creates a protective "halo" around the damaged tooth root, this inhibits the dentist's anesthetic from working effectively. After forty-eight to seventy-two hours of antibiotic regimen, the patient will return to the dentist to resume treatment, which can now progress comfortably.

If there is damage to the tooth nerve and pulp, a root-canal procedure will be used to remove the infection and decay from the root area. When this treatment is complete, a porcelain or gold crown is fabricated to restore the tooth to its ideal form and function.

WHAT TO DO

- Trapped food particles between teeth may cause or contribute to tooth pain. Use dental floss to remove any food gently. Rinse with a warm salt-water mixture.
- Avoid exercise for the duration of the pain.
- For tooth infection and resulting pain, place ice or a cold can of soda over the cheek on the affected side for no more than 15 minutes of each hour.
- Moisten a cotton ball with oil of cloves and apply to the damaged tooth with tweezers.
- Avoid flying and scuba diving. Both may increase pressure on the damaged tooth.
- Prevent future tooth problems by brushing and flossing regularly after meals and having teeth professionally examined and cleaned regularly.
- Wear protective equipment and mouth guards when playing sports.

The Respiratory System

GENERAL INFORMATION

The respiratory system, consisting of the nose, throat, windpipe (trachea), and lungs, filters and warms air for the circulatory system.

Tiny hairs and mucus in the nose prevent most microscopic particles from reaching the lungs. The air passes through the larynx, into the trachea, and then into the lungs. When viruses attack the respiratory system, the nose and trachea are usually the initial sites of infection. Coughing or sneezing spreads infections to other sites.

RESPIRATORY SPECIALISTS

PRIMARY-CARE PHYSICIAN (M.D.). An internist trained in internal medicine or a family practitioner/pediatrician.

OTOLARYNGOLOGIST (M.D.). An otolaryngologist is trained medically and surgically to treat disorders of the ear, nose, throat, head, and neck. Often called an ear, nose, and throat (ENT) specialist, this doctor is certified by the American Board of Otolaryngology–Head and Neck Surgery.

ALLERGIST (M.D.). A physician with additional training in diagnosing and treating allergic disease, certified by the American Board of Allergy and Immunology.

PULMONOLOGIST (M.D.). An internist or pediatrician with additional training in diagnosing and treating diseases of the lungs.

PHYSICIAN'S CARE REQUIRED

ASTHMA. Chronic breathing disorder characterized by shortness of breath, wheezing, and tightness in chest. Triggered by allergens, exercise, cold air, respiratory

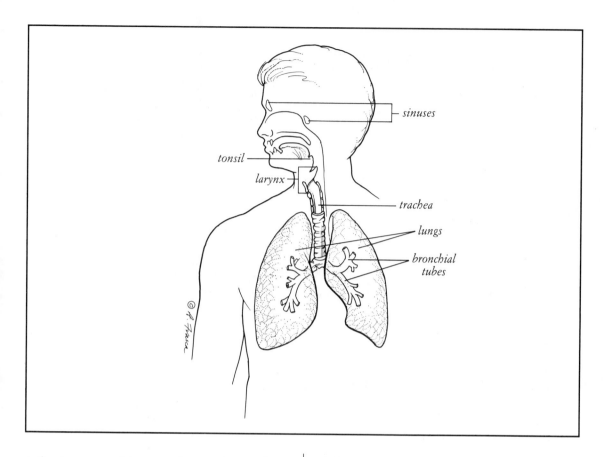

sinuses

tonsil

larynx

trachea

lungs

bronchial tubes

infections, smoking, and certain medications. An allergy specialist will examine, point out probable causes, and treat with a variety of medications, including powerful inhaled drugs.

BRONCHITIS. Inflammation of the bronchi, the main air passages of the lungs, characterized by pain in the upper chest area and back, and a wheezing, deep cough that brings up yellow or gray phlegm from the lungs. Bronchitis is typically caused by a virus, so no specific treatment is possible. Doctor may prescribe a cough suppressant or bronchodilator medications.

EMPHYSEMA. Chronic, incurable lung disease caused by smoking, genetic defect, air pollution, or injury to the chest; characterized by a shortness of breath that worsens over time and a barrel-like chest deformity. Prescription medications plus giving up smoking may slow the progress of the disease.

PNEUMONIA. Bacterial or viral-induced lung inflammation. Symptoms include high fever, chills, cough (with or without bloody sputum), rapid breathing, and fatigue. Doctor may take chest X ray and blood sample. If the pneumonia is bacterial, medication is prescribed, but no specific treatment is available for viral pneumonia.

continued on page 115

COMMON RESPIRATORY PROBLEMS

COLD
A common, virus-related illness typified by low-grade fever, nasal congestion, watery eyes, cough and/or headache. Nasal decongestants can help in symptomatic relief. **Page 115**

COUGH
A symptom that indicates that the throat, larynx, bronchial tubes, or lungs are irritated or infected. A cough is an effort to remove the irritating substance. **Page 118**

FLU
Common symptoms of cough, sore throat, headache, muscle aches and pains, fever, and fatigue call for bed rest. No cure, but annual flu shots prevent lung infections and the more dangerous pneumonia. This is especially important for people with decreased resistance to infection, such as the elderly or immune compromised. **Page 120**

HAY FEVER
Common seasonal or year-round allergic reaction to various allergens. Hay fever can't be cured, but many self-help measures and medications can greatly reduce symptoms. **Page 122**

LARYNGITIS
An irritation or inflammation of the vocal cords through voice abuse, bacterial or viral infection, or inhalation of caustic fumes. **Page 126**

SORE THROAT
Pain in the throat is a symptom of an infection or an irritation of the pharynx, the back area of the mouth beyond the tongue. Pain symptoms can be relieved with self-help measures. **Page 128**

TUBERCULOSIS. TB is an infectious bacterial disease that attacks the lungs and is transmitted through the air from one person to another via cough or sneeze. Symptoms are not apparent early. Weight loss, night sweats, fatigue, and/or a dry hacking cough that produces bloody or pus-filled phlegm begin months to years after exposure. Doctor will examine and prescribe medication and antibiotics to cure. TB vaccines are available for high-risk individuals.

COLD

Kathleen L. Yaremchuk, M.D.

Dr. Yaremchuk is clinical professor of Otolaryngology at the University of Michigan Medical School, and senior staff member of the Department of Otolaryngology, Henry Ford Hospital, Detroit, Michigan

The common cold is a temporary, self-limiting upper-respiratory viral infection that affects the nose and throat. It can strike at any time of the year. More than 200 different viruses cause cold symptoms.

As a rule, colds last five to seven days, but may linger for two weeks. Typical symptoms include a congested or runny nose with clear mucus; a sore, scratchy throat; hoarseness; coughing; watery eyes; sneezing; muscle aches and pain; and headache.

A cold can often be mistaken for the flu (see FLU, page 120), but high temperatures, body aches and pains, and a deep fatigue typically separates the flu from a cold. With a cold, oral body temperature is usually in the 99 degree range.

Colds, which are easily spread by finger touch, are most prevalent from September through May, when people spend more time indoors. Children are more susceptible to colds because they haven't built up appropriate antibodies to the different cold viruses, and spend much time in classrooms, where close contact facilitates viral transmissions. When a cold hits a child, lymph glands in the neck may swell and become tender, and fever may approach 103 degrees F. Children typically get up to eight colds each year, adults many fewer— one cold per year on average by the age of sixty.

Treatment

Since a cold is a viral infection, antibiotics are of no use in symptomatic treatment. However, OTC cold remedies including cough syrups, cough drops, decongestants, pain relievers, and combination cold medicines can help the symptoms. Whenever I or someone in my family develops a cold, I make use of them very quickly. I jump on a cold at its first symptom, because I've found that a day or two of early intervention can relieve symptoms and help keep the cold from turning into something worse.

When the nose becomes congested, the swelling of the nasal lining closes the sinuses. When the sinuses can't drain, they can become infected and turn a common cold into a sinus or middle ear infection that requires a doctor's immediate attention.

If you don't have high blood pressure, diabetes, heart disease, or any other medical problem, nasal decongestants can be a great help for a cold. Available OTC in the pharmacy as pills, nose drops, or inhaled preparations, decongestants work by constricting the blood vessels in the nose, which temporarily opens the nasal passages, preventing the sinuses from being blocked. You also feel better because you no longer have to breathe through your mouth.

In the first three or four days of a cold, nasal spray decongestants can be effective. The one drawback is the rebound phenomenon that can occur after they have been used for more than five days. The congestion and accompanying swelling comes back as bad as before or even worse, and the medication spray becomes ineffective for treatment. Therefore, only use decongestants for four days. Let nature do the rest.

Another big help is a humidifier. From the time the heat goes on in the house in the fall until it goes off in the spring, my house is dry, which predisposes my family and me to upper respiratory infections. A humidifier helps reduce the chance. If you do come down with a cold, place a humidifier in the room. The increased water in the air helps keep your sinuses moist, which helps loosen any mucus secretions that have built up.

Mild exercise helps relieve cold symptoms, because it acts as a natural decongestant by increasing adrenaline, which leads to increased air flow through the nose. The release of endorphins—the body's natural opiates—which occurs during exercise will also make you feel a little better as well.

However, don't take the "little is good, so more is better" approach and try to put yourself through a normal or above-average workout when you have a cold. Asking your body to exercise strenuously while fighting cold symptoms at the same time may be too much, and you may actually worsen your symptoms. Listen to your body. If you don't feel too well, just go for a brief walk and then head home. Or take a break from your workouts, and don't do anything at all.

If your cold is accompanied by high fever and/or vomiting, this can lead to mild dehydration, so water intake has to be increased at this time. Don't exercise when you have these additional symptoms. You can worsen an already difficult situation.

Drink a lot of fluids. This means 8 cups a day. It will help keep your respiratory tract moist and replace any fluids lost through elevated temperature.

Adequate rest certainly helps you feel better. If you don't feel well, stay home from work. If you don't take time to rest, you may pay for it by delaying recovery and not performing up to par. You also expose others to the infection by going to work.

To relieve muscular aches and pains that accompany a cold, take ibuprofen or acetaminophen. Aspirin is not recommended for anyone under nineteen years of age because of its link with Reye's syndrome, a potentially dangerous, sometimes fatal disorder.

To relieve sore throat symptoms that accompany a cold, gargle with warm salt water. (Add 1 teaspoon of salt to 1 quart of warm water.)

Hot liquids are also beneficial. Chicken soup has long been touted as a cold remedy. In one Florida study it was found that the hot steam coming off the soup helps to open the nasal passages temporarily. If you don't like chicken soup, try your favorite soup or clear, hot beverage instead.

Prevention

- To decrease your chances of getting a cold, keep your fingers away from your eyes, nose, and mouth.
- Wash your hands regularly throughout the day with warm water and soap to kill the viruses.
- Avoid using the belongings of a person with a cold, such as soap, tools, drinking glasses, or even the telephone.

Cause for Concern

If your cold symptoms last longer than five days and seem to be worsening, or if you have a fever over 103 degrees F that lasts for two days, see your doctor. The same advice holds if you develop severe chest and head pains, or if the color of your sputum changes from clear to yellow or brown and remains that way for several days, or if you develop an earache. These are signs your common cold may have developed into a bacterial infection, which can be treated with antibiotics.

WHAT TO DO

- Keep your fingers away from your nose, eyes, and mouth.

- Wash your hands regularly throughout the day with warm water and soap to kill the cold virus.
- Avoid using the belongings of a person with a cold. Be especially careful of toys that may be shared by children.
- Use nasal decongestants to open sinuses if you have no history of high blood pressure.
- Use a humidifier in cold weather months to keep the upper respiratory tract moist. This increases the natural cleansing action of nose and sinuses and prevents nosebleeds.
- Light exercise helps relieve cold symptoms. Don't push yourself and go too hard or symptoms may worsen.
- Dress warmly, keep up fluid intake, and get adequate rest.
- For relief of muscular aches and pains, take acetaminophen or ibuprofen. Children under nineteen should not take aspirin because of its link with Reye's syndrome.
- Gargle with a warm salt-water solution to relieve sore-throat symptoms.
- If cold symptoms worsen and last longer than five days, if you develop an earache, or have a fever over 103 degrees F that lasts for two days, or have severe chest or head pains, contact your physician.

COUGH

Edward R. Garrity, Jr., M.D.

*Dr. Garrity is director of the Pulmonary Function Laboratory at the
Loyola University Medical Center in Maywood, Illinois*

A cough is a response to irritation in the throat, larynx, bronchial tubes, or lungs. There are two distinct types of coughs, productive and nonproductive. A productive cough brings up sputum from the respiratory tract, which is necessary for recovery.

A nonproductive cough is dry and scratchy and raises no sputum. Nonproductive coughs are often caused by the common cold or flu, asthma, dust, an object or piece of food trapped in the airways, pollution, and cigarette smoke.

The sound your cough makes can be an indicator of its source. A barking cough could suggest bronchitis, an infection of the bronchial tubes. Sometimes it could mean croup, a common illness in children under three years of age, which is caused by a cold virus. A high-pitched cough can mean the vocal cords are involved and the airways have become narrowed. A wheezing sound often indicates asthma, bronchitis, or both. Loud, gasping coughing points to pertussis, commonly called whooping cough, a severe infection of the respiratory tract, highly contagious.

Treatment

A cough is most often caused by the common cold, and typically it runs its course in two weeks or less without treatment. If the cold-induced cough is productive and brings up collected mucus from the respiratory tract, don't limit or stop this with cough suppressant medications. However, you may want to loosen thick mucus to make it easier to get out of the lungs. Many people use expectorant medications to do this. I feel OTC cough medicines containing an expectorant such as guaifenesin—a drug that is supposed to loosen mucus—are generally ineffective.

To loosen mucus, I recommend drinking plenty of water, fruit juice, carbonated beverages, or hot tea. The liquids provide extra moisture to help loosen and thin out the mucus. Take a hot bath or shower and inhale the thick clouds of steam to loosen the congestion.

If you have a winter cough and your home is dry and overheated, use a vaporizer in your room to add moisture to the dry air. This is especially important at night when you sleep. Humidified air helps liquefy the mucus and makes your cough more productive. One word of caution: vaporizers can harbor bacteria and fungi that can aggravate or even cause a cough. Be sure to clean your machine regularly and keep it properly maintained.

If I have a cold accompanied by a cough, I generally let the cold run its course without doing anything specific to limit the cough. However, if I have an unproductive, dry, hacking cough that lingers beyond all other cold symptoms—a common occurrence—I will take an OTC medicine containing the cough suppressant dextromethorphan.

Dextromethorphan, an FDA-approved

nonprescription antitussive drug, acts to suppress the part of the brain that controls the cough reflex. Although in most cases it won't stop a cough completely, it can limit it and make you more comfortable. Cough suppressants are for short-term use and generally should be stopped after three days.

Cough drops you buy in candy stores and supermarkets coat the mouth with saliva and make it feel better by temporarily breaking the cough cycle. However, there's no medicine in cough drops, and sucking on a piece of hard candy will yield the same results.

Cause for Concern

If coughing brings up mucus that is yellow, brown, or green, it may indicate infection that needs to be treated by a doctor. If the mucus is blood-tinged or bright red in color, contact your doctor immediately. Excessive coughing itself can cause blood vessels in the throat to rupture and bleed, which is not a serious problem. However, you may have an acute respiratory ailment that causes bleeding, and this needs to be treated immediately. To be sure, don't self-diagnose. Let the doctor examine you.

If you don't smoke and have healthy lungs, you will rarely cough, and if coughing is triggered by a common cold or flu, it should clear up within ten to fourteen days. However, contact your family doctor if you cough for more than three days for no obvious reason, or have a cough that doesn't get better within two weeks. Remember, a persistent cough is a telling symptom for a number of serious diseases. You should also consult your doctor if coughing is accompanied by a fever, skin rash, thick sputum, an earache, chest pain, shortness of breath, lethargy, pain in the teeth or sinuses, or confusion.

What the Doctor Will Do

After taking your medical history, the doctor may x-ray your chest and sinuses, take a culture of your sputum, and prescribe appropriate medication. If it's warranted, you will be sent to a medical specialist to treat the underlying illness causing your cough.

WHAT TO DO

- Drink plenty of water, fruit juice, carbonated beverages, or hot tea to keep the airways moist.
- Inhale the steam from a hot bath or shower, or inhale the vapor from a boiling pan of water.
- Use a vaporizer in your room, especially at night when sleeping. Keep the vaporizer very clean.
- Don't use cough syrup containing expectorant medication. They are ineffective.

To stop an unproductive, dry, hacking cough that interferes with daily activity and sleep:

- Use a cough syrup containing dextromethorphan according to directions, but for no more than three days.
- Suck on a cough drop or piece of candy.
- Contact your family doctor if your cough lasts longer than three days for unexplained reasons, or if it is accompanied by a headache, fever, chest pain, shortness of breath, or thick brown, green, yellow, or red mucus.

FLU

Parker A. Small, Jr., M.D.

*Dr. Small is professor of Immunology and Medical Microbiology and professor of Pediatrics
at the University of Florida College of Medicine, Gainesville*

Influenza, more commonly known as flu, is a viral infection that infects one in four Americans each winter. It's also the sixth leading cause of death in this country, killing 40,000 to 50,000 annually. Those at greatest risk are the elderly, pregnant women, cancer patients, and people with heart disease or respiratory illness.

The flu virus has been around for centuries, and it is among the fastest changing viruses. New strains develop about every ten years, and milder changes occur every year. Flu viruses emerge when animal viruses hook together with human counterparts, forming a completely different virus. The viruses are often given names based on their place of origin, for example, the Asian flu.

The flu virus is spread through the air by sneezing or coughing. In this age of international travel, airplanes, which use recirculated air in the cabin, are the major transporters of flu around the globe.

Flu typically strikes in the fall, peaks during winter, and begins to fade as summer approaches. Symptoms develop within seventy-two hours after exposure and include fever up to 104 degrees that can last for three to five days, a dry cough, sore throat, headache, joint pain, chills, and a burning sensation in the eyes. If the flu spreads from the upper respiratory tract to the lungs, secondary bacterial pneumonia can develop. It's virtually impossible to tell the difference between a mild flu and a cold (see COLD, page 115). However, if you come down with symptoms at the same time that a flu epidemic is present in your community, it's likely that you have the flu as well.

Prevention

- A flu shot is usually effective for at least a year, and can be life saving for the elderly, and for people with chronic lung disease, chronic heart disease, or other serious illnesses. It generally takes up to two weeks to induce substantial immunity, and should be given between September and November each year, well before the flu season begins. If you have a proven allergy to eggs, don't get a flu shot. The vaccine is made with an egg base and could trigger an adverse reaction.

- Amantadine, a prescription antiviral medication, can be taken in place of a flu shot. Effective against type A flu virus but not type B, amantadine will prevent infection, or if used early in the course of flu infection, can reduce the severity of the disease.

Treatment

Flu is a viral infection and antibiotics are not effective against it. However, if you're not in a risk group that is susceptible to flu complications, you can treat yourself successfully at home. The symptomatic approach passed on by generations of mothers and grandmothers—rest, keep warm, drink plenty of fluids—is still the best medicine.

The overriding goal in flu treatment is to keep the virus out of the lungs. Stay in bed until your temperature returns to normal and you no longer have body aches and pains. If you go to work or try to exercise in the misguided belief that you can work or run through your sickness, you will breathe harder and likely move the virus from the upper to the lower respiratory tract. Remember: vigorous activity has the potential to make flu much worse.

Drink fluids. It doesn't matter if they are cold or hot as long as you drink at least 8 cups a day. Fluids prevent dehydration and keep the protective mucous lining of the respiratory system moist and intact so it can effectively fight off the virus.

Keep warm. Staying warm helps prevent the flu virus from growing. If you go outside and breathe in cold air, you lower the surface temperature of the nose and trachea, and this helps encourage flu growth.

For the average child or adult, a fever of up to 102 degrees F acts as an antiviral agent. You shouldn't take acetaminophen or ibuprofen to try to lower your fever if you're in that range.

However, if your fever reaches 103 degrees F or higher, take two acetaminophen or ibuprofen every four hours. Aspirin should *never* be taken if you are nineteen or younger because of its association with Reye's syndrome.

Vitamin C is a controversial topic. Some studies indicate that 500 milligrams of vitamin C four times daily help minimize flu symptoms, while other studies show no benefit whatsoever. At this dosage, it does no harm.

There is also a debate within the medical community about the use of OTC cough preparations for relief of cough symptoms that accompany a flu. Many pulmonologists are against their use, because the cough acts to clean and move matter from the lungs. Although in general I agree with this approach, I usually modify it for the flu. Classically, a flu infection produces a dry, hacking cough, which is unproductive and does not help recovery. In addition to irritating the lining of the throat, it can spread the virus down into the lungs.

With the unproductive cough of a flu, use an OTC cough suppressant, or antitussive, containing dextromethorphan. This derivative of morphine won't make you drowsy or nauseate you. It inhibits coughing by affecting the cough reflex in the brain. It can also be used during the day as needed, and also at night to assure better sleep.

My one caveat: Do not use cough medicine the first two hours after awaking in the morning, because if there is a buildup of sputum in the lungs, you need to cough to bring it up and out.

Cause for Concern

The minute you see green or yellow sputum, stop all cough suppressants. Pus in the lungs indicates an infection, and the only way to get it out is by coughing it out. Contact your physician immediately for an examination.

Your doctor should also be contacted if you are not feeling any better by day 5 of your flu, or if you start to feel better and then suffer a relapse. This is typical of a bacterial lung infection.

Also, contact your doctor if you have chest pain, fatigue, or hoarseness. These are also indications of a bacterial super-infection, and you need to be treated with doctor-prescribed antibiotics.

REYE'S SYNDROME

Reye's syndrome, a rare, but fast-progressing and often fatal childhood disorder, can develop as a child recovers from the flu. If your child becomes drowsy, begins to vomit, or hallucinates after having the flu, contact your doctor immediately. Do not give aspirin. There is a deadly link, not yet fully understood, between aspirin and Reye's syndrome.

WHAT TO DO

- Stay in bed until temperature returns to normal.
- Keep warm.
- Drink 8 cups of fluid a day.
- Don't routinely treat a fever of up to 102 degrees F with acetaminophen or ibuprofen. The fever *helps* fight the virus.
- Take acetaminophen or ibuprofen for muscular aches and pains, or fever higher than 102 degrees F.
- Don't give aspirin to children because of its link to Reye's syndrome.
- Use cough suppressants as needed to suppress dry, nonproductive coughs. Don't use them in the morning until congestion collected in the chest overnight is first coughed up.
- Have an annual flu shot.
- If you cough up green or yellow sputum, have chest pain or hoarseness, or start to get better and then suddenly feel worse, contact your physician. These are signs of a bacterial lung infection and need to be promptly treated.

HAY FEVER

Sidney Friedlaender, M.D.

Dr. Friedlaender is clinical professor of medicine at the University of Florida, in Gainesville, and editor-in-chief of Immunology and Allergy Practice Journal

Hay fever, or allergic rhinitis, has nothing to do with hay, and rarely does it cause a fever. It was named by a nineteenth-century English doctor who developed an allergic reaction in his nose and eyes when he ventured into a hay barn. It was later discovered that his allergy was to a mold in the barn, but the name hay fever has stuck ever since.

For more than 35 million Americans who come into seasonal contact with airborne pollens from budding trees, shrubs, grasses, and flowers, abnormal physical reactions are triggered in the upper respiratory tract. Sneezing, runny nose, congestion, scratchy throat, wheezing, and itchy, watery eyes are the most common symptoms.

These allergic reactions are caused when the body's immune defense overreacts to these substances. Allergy antibodies exist in everyone. When an allergen such as tree pollen comes into contact with a specific tree-pollen antibody in an allergic person, histamines and other chemical substances called mediators are released. Sneezing, watery eyes, and congestion soon follow.

Allergy symptoms are similar to those of the common cold. But with hay fever, nasal secretion is watery and thin, not thick, yellow, and mucusy like a cold.

You may suspect you have an allergy if you experience the same adverse reactions each year at about the same time, or if at least 10 percent of the people in your community experience the same reaction. Allergies are the most common in spring and fall, but some people have allergies year-round. These are typically caused by molds, mildew, and microscopic dust mites that are found in the cleanest homes, and animal hair dander, especially from cats.

The hay fever season varies according to where you live. In southern states, it's common in January and February, when local trees begin to blossom, and continues straight through to autumn, with grasses and flower pollen, and finally ragweed, a principal cause of hay fever for many people.

In the Northeast and Midwest, it begins in March when trees start pollinating, and ends usually in early autumn when the ragweed dies off. The northwest part of the country doesn't have a major ragweed problem, but the grasses pollinate for half the year, extending the allergy season from March through early December. In the Rocky Mountain states, the allergy season is from April to October.

Weather strongly affects allergies. Cool or rainy days will keep pollen levels down, while hot, windy days will cause pollen levels to rise dramatically.

Treatment

There is no cure for hay fever, but knowing your allergic "trigger" and taking appropriate measures to minimize it is the best treatment. Discovering specifically what causes your allergy is a big first step.

Be aware of pollen and mold levels in your area. Check your local newspaper, radio, and television weather broadcasts before heading outdoors.

If you start sneezing when you begin cutting your lawn, then grass is probably your allergic trigger. Keep your lawn cut as short as possible so the grass won't bloom. Wear a surgical mask that covers the mouth and nose when you mow your lawn to keep pollens out of your respiratory system. These masks are available in the local pharmacy. Don't reuse a mask, because it gets covered with pollen. If a walk in the woods causes allergic symptoms, or if they coincide with a high ragweed count, then trees or ragweed may be the troublemakers.

If you are in the midst of your allergy "season," take your medication—either OTC or prescription—30 minutes before going outdoors. It takes that much time to be absorbed. Avoid exercising in the morning between 5 and 10, when plants produce the most pollen. Instead, exercise later in the day, when pollen levels taper off. Swimming is an excellent aerobic conditioner that reduces your contact with airborne allergens.

With the window open, run your car's air conditioner for several minutes before you get in. This gets rid of pollen or mold that may have collected in the cooling system. When driving, keep the windows up, and use the air conditioner if needed.

Wear sunglasses not just for protection from harmful sun rays, but to keep the airborne pollens from getting in your eyes.

If you are highly allergic, after being outside for an extended period, take a shower to wash pollens from hair and skin. Rinse your eyes with cool water to clear any clinging allergens. If you are able to wear contact lenses during your allergy season, be sure to rinse them off with your saline solution to dislodge any pollen.

If you have year-round allergies, keep your house as pollen-free as possible. Switch to special allergen-proof covers for your box springs, mattresses, and pillowcases. Don't store anything under your bed because this can harbor pollen, dust, and dust mites.

Replace your woolen blankets with blankets of either cotton or man-made fabrics. If you use a comforter, make sure it's filled with a synthetic fiber and not goose down.

Install special high-efficiency electronic filters in your home air-conditioning and heating units to help reduce the amount of circulating pollen and dust in the house.

Vacuum your home regularly, but vacuum your bedroom daily. A single speck of dust contains a mix of fabric fibers, mold spores, animal dander if you have a pet, and dust mites. If possible, don't keep a rug in your room. It's a trap for allergens. If you have wooden floors, mopping is the best way to get up the dust. If you vacuum, use a hard canister vacuum with a filter. After vacuuming anywhere in the house, avoid the area for at least two hours to let any allergens settle back down on the ground.

Instead of heavy draperies or Venetian blinds, switch to roller shades or washable curtains in your bedroom. Keep all books out of the bedroom. They are great dust collectors.

Dander, the microscopic flakes of skin from cats, dogs, rabbits, hamsters, gerbils, and birds, all can cause allergic reactions, as can the saliva from some animals. If you can't part with your pet, then limit its range to just one or two rooms in the house, and make your bedroom off-limits. When it's time to clean your pet, have someone in the family do it who's not allergic. Bathing will clean the fur of dander, saliva, and pollens. A bimonthly rinse of 1 teaspoonful of fabric softener added to 1 quart of water—which is safe for your animal—will cut down static electricity on the animal's coat, and help reduce the number of allergens clinging to it. When your pet comes indoors after a walk or extended stay outdoors, run a damp cloth over the coat to remove all collected pollens.

To cut down on mold growth, don't use wallpaper on kitchen or bathroom walls. If you replace the wallpaper, use mold-proof paint in its place.

If your house is particularly damp, use a dehumidifier and be sure to change and clean the water receptacle regularly to prevent mold growth.

At night, keep windows closed and use the air conditioner, which cleans, cools, and dries the air, filtering out offending pollens. Clean the air filter regularly. Central air-conditioning in the home can dramatically reduce allergens. If you have severe allergy problems and can afford it, central air will quickly pay dividends.

Don't smoke and make it a point to

avoid those who do. Tobacco smoke aggravates the nasal passages.

Medications

If you have a mild, seasonal hay fever lasting three to fourteen days, buy one of the more popular OTC hay fever remedies such as Chlor-Trimeton or Benadryl. These antihistamines are effective and safe.

Check the OTC antihistamine labels carefully. The effective medications contain a high percentage of chlorpheniramine —anywhere from 4 mg to 8 mg. Chlorpheniramine is the gold standard and is available in more than half of the OTC products sold. It has a forty-year record of safety and effectiveness.

Many OTC medications have a sedating side effect on some people. The effect depends on your age (children under twelve may become quite drowsy), your weight (people 100 pounds or less may become drowsy), and your metabolism (if your system doesn't metabolize medications quickly, you may feel tired). Therefore, in some cases a medication with only 4 mg of chlorpheniramine may actually work better for you than one containing 8 mg. The only way to find out is to try one.

If the medication makes you tired or sluggish, stay with the drug for five to seven days, but start with one-fourth or one-half the recommended dosage and increase it over the next few days to the full dosage. Take your medication in the morning, at least a half hour before you plan to go out. This gives the medication plenty of time to work in your system.

If your child has allergic symptoms, consult with your physician before giving any OTC medications. The incidence of asthma in children, a chronic, obstructive disorder of the airways often triggered by allergies, is so high that a pediatrician or allergist needs to diagnose the problem.

What the Doctor Will Do

If OTC allergy medications prove ineffective, contact a board-certified allergist. The doctor will take a history to make the right diagnosis. To find out specifically what you're allergic to, you'll be given a "prick" skin test in which various allergens are injected just below the skin, or a RAST (radioallergosorbent) test, in which blood is taken and analyzed for allergy antibodies. Appropriate medication will then be prescribed.

The more popular medications include terfenadine tablets, which inhibit allergy symptoms without causing drowsiness, cromolyn sodium nasal spray and eye drops, which are not good for onetime acute cases, but, when used regularly, build up in the system and are very effective. Flunisolide and beclomethasone dipropionate nasal sprays are also widely used. All of these steroidal mixtures are effective in reducing mucus production and shrinking swollen nasal passages.

If you can't get relief from OTC medication or from prescription drugs, or if you feel your allergies are an impediment to your life-style, the allergist might recommend that you begin immunotherapy. This is also known as desensitization shots, or more commonly as "allergy shots."

In some instances, immunotherapy can be very effective. Injections are taken weekly for at least three to five years, with allergic symptoms usually subsiding after one to two years. The shots don't contain medication, but rather a carefully selected and purified extract of the pollens that cause you problems. In theory, your body builds up tolerance to the injected substances, and when you do come into contact with the offending pollen, there will be little or no reaction. If you see no benefit after three years, you should stop taking the shots.

WHAT TO DO

- Keep your lawn cut as short as possible to prevent the grass from blooming.
- Avoid exercising in the early morning hours.
- When driving, keep the windows up and use the air conditioner if needed.
- After being outside for extended periods, take a shower to wash off pollen from hair and skin.
- For year-round allergies, keep your house as pollen-free as possible.

- Switch to allergen-proof covers for box springs, mattresses, and pillowcases.
- Replace woolen blankets with cotton or synthetics.
- Vacuum your bedroom daily.
- Keep all books out of the bedroom.
- Limit your pet's range to one or two rooms in the house. Keep the bedroom off-limits.
- Don't use wallpaper on the kitchen or bathroom walls if you're allergic to mold. Use mold-proof paint in its place.
- Keep windows closed in the house and use air-conditioning.
- Use high-efficiency electronic filters in air-conditioning and heating systems.
- Don't smoke.
- If you have mild, seasonal hay fever lasting three to fourteen days, use OTC antihistamine medications containing chlorpheniramine as directed.
- If OTC medications are ineffective, contact a board-certified allergist for allergy testing and possible immunotherapy, which could result in long-term relief.

LARYNGITIS

Michael S. Benninger, M.D.

Dr. Benninger is vice-chairman, Department of Otolaryngology–Head and Neck Surgery at the Henry Ford Hospital in Detroit, Michigan

Laryngitis is either a viral or bacterial inflammation of the vocal cords (the larynx), which is located at the top of the windpipe. Swelling of the larynx causes the major symptom of the ailment, which is a hoarse, husky, or raspy voice. In some advanced cases, speaking becomes impossible. Laryngitis is rarely serious and typically lasts a week or so, but longer if you abuse your voice in the meantime.

If children develop laryngitis, complications can arise because the opening of a child's larynx is so small. Swelling may cause problems with breathing or swallowing. If this occurs, contact your physician immediately.

The most common cause of laryngitis is voice abuse, such as excessive singing, singing in the wrong pitch, or singing music that stresses the larynx. Talking too much can also bring about laryngitis, as can screaming and smoking. The throat becomes inflamed, the larynx swells, and the vocal cords don't vibrate normally. Your voice becomes low, deep, and breathy.

Treatment

If you have an uncomplicated case of laryngitis, several things will ease the symptoms until the condition clears. A rule of thumb is not to speak to anyone that you cannot touch. Having to raise your voice strains the vocal cords even more.

Minimize the use of your voice. If the laryngitis is severe, don't talk at all.

Don't whisper. Whispering is actually harder on the larynx than gentle, confidential-level speech. Speak only in a slightly breathy manner, but not in a whisper. If possible, write notes instead of talking.

Drink plenty of warm fluids to keep the larynx moist. Too cold or hot liquids may be irritating to the throat. Stay away from caffeinated beverages. Caffeine is a diuretic and tends to decrease moisture. Avoid milk; although there is no hard evidence to support it, milk and milk products may tend to thicken the mucus in the throat, which adds to hoarseness. Drink water or noncitric juice such as grape or apple juice instead.

To help moisturize the larynx, squeeze a slice of lemon into room-temperature water and drink it.

Gargling with warm, slightly salted water can also stimulate saliva flow, making the throat feel more comfortable.

To moisturize the larynx directly, spray the back of the throat with warm salt water in a fine-spray mister.

Many homes are kept too hot and dry in the winter. A cool-mist vaporizer, especially in the bedroom at night, will help put water back into the air and relieve sore throat and laryngitis symptoms. Remember to keep these devices clean and use filters when needed.

Don't smoke. In addition to increasing your cancer risk, smoking can cause laryngitis as well as aggravate an existing case.

Avoid alcoholic beverages. Alcohol leads to dryness and numbs the vocal cords so you don't realize you're hurting them when you speak.

Clear your throat only when necessary. Throat clearing hurts and irritates the throat. When you feel the urge to clear your throat, swallow warm water instead. This will help remove the accumulated mucus and soothe the throat.

Contact a voice coach or speech language pathologist if you are a person who uses either your singing or speaking voice for a living. You will be taught techniques for appropriate voice use without irritation.

Cause for Concern

If you have laryngitis, accompanied by a persistent cough that continues for more than three to four weeks, or if you have recurrent laryngitis, contact an otolaryngologist (an ENT: an ear, nose, and throat specialist) for a complete exam. More severe illnesses are occasionally masked by laryngitis.

What the Doctor Will Do

If laryngitis continues for more than a week after following these home measures, contact your primary-care physician. He'll check the back of the throat for typical symptoms of acute infection, and listen to the lungs for signs of congestion. If a bacterial infection is the cause of laryngitis, antibiotics will be prescribed.

WHAT TO DO

- Don't speak to anyone you can't touch.
- Decrease amount of talking. Determine amount by level of discomfort.
- Don't whisper when you have to talk. Speak in slightly breathy tones.
- If possible, write notes instead of talking.
- Drink plenty of warm, body-temperature fluids.

- Don't drink caffeinated beverages.
- Milk may thicken mucus in the throat. Drink water or grape and apple fruit juice instead.
- Squeeze a lemon slice into warm water and drink it.
- Spray the back of the throat with warm saline water in a fine-spray mister.
- Use a cool-mist vaporizer, especially in the bedroom.
- Don't smoke.
- Don't drink alcoholic beverages.
- Don't clear your throat excessively. Swallow warm water instead to remove accumulated mucus.
- If you use either your singing or speaking voice for a living, a voice coach or speech language pathologist will be able to teach you techniques for appropriate voice use without irritation.
- If laryngitis continues for more than a week, or you have difficulty breathing or swallowing, contact your physician.

SORE THROAT

Steven J. Pearlman, M.D.

Dr. Pearlman is associate director of the Department of Otolaryngology at the St. Luke's/Roosevelt Hospital Center in New York City

A sore throat, or acute pharyngitis, is one of the most common winter complaints. It is a symptom of an infection —usually viral—or an irritation of the pharynx, the back column of the mouth behind the tongue. Irritation may be a local throat infection or result from post nasal drip due to discharge from allergic reaction, sinusitis, or a head cold.

Children are especially susceptible to sore throats because their immune systems aren't mature enough to fend off the cold and flu viruses. They are also frequently bombarded with viruses from sneezing and coughing classmates.

Sore throats caused by a cold or flu virus (see COLD, page 115; FLU, page 120) are usually self-limiting, and will clear on their own in a few days. They don't respond to antibiotics, but symptoms can be diminished with self-help measures.

The 10 to 15 percent of sore throats caused by bacterial infections, either streptococcus (strep throat) or staphylococcus bacteria, should be treated with doctor-prescribed antibiotics, rest, self-treatment, or all three.

Without a throat culture, it's difficult to differentiate a viral sore throat from one caused by bacteria. However, sore throats caused by a virus develop gradually over a period of time. They are often accompanied by the flu or cold, and if a fever is present, it will generally be in the range of 101 degrees F or below.

A bacterial sore throat usually comes on fast, lymph glands of the neck often swell and become tender, and a headache develops (see HEADACHE, page 219). Fever is typically 102 degrees F or higher. The throat may appear extremely red and have either white or yellow spots at the back.

Treatment

To relieve sore throat pain, follow the same time-honored theory used in treating a cold: good nutrition, adequate rest, chicken soup, and plenty of liquids. (In addition, I use my own personal remedy, which is to suck Callard & Bowser butterscotch candy throughout the day. Although these candies don't kill any throat germs, they increase the production of saliva and soothe my raspy, painful throat.)

Many OTC lozenges, some of which contain mild anesthetics, also provide temporary relief for sore throat symptoms. Gargling several times a day with a mixture of 1 teaspoon of salt stirred into 8 ounces of warm water can also temporarily soothe a sore throat, break up congestion, and help flush out bacteria. A cup of tea can relieve a sore throat by warming the irritated membranes.

Use a humidifier or a cool-mist vaporizer in your bedroom at night to add extra moisture to the air and keep your nasal membranes and throat lining moist. Cool-air vaporizers have gotten some bad press because improperly maintained machines can send dust mites and mold spores all over a room. In the case of ultrasonic humidifiers, they can coat furniture with a fine, white film. This can trigger allergies, colds, flu, and sore throats. However, if you clean the water tank according to instructions, these machines will help alleviate more health problems than they cause.

People with cold-congested noses tend to breathe through their mouths. This dries out the throat and makes it sore. Drink extra liquids throughout the day to prevent it.

OTC nasal sprays may also be helpful, but do not use them for more than three days because you may suffer from the "rebound effect." Mucus production may be temporarily halted by the nasal spray, but as the body builds a tolerance, these sprays lose effectiveness, and mucus secretion increases dramatically, raising the level of nasal discomfort.

To help relieve the pain and inflammation of a sore throat, take 2 aspirin, acetaminophen, or ibuprofen tablets every four hours. Children should not take aspirin because of its link with Reye's syndrome, a potentially life-threatening disorder.

Cause for Concern

See a doctor immediately if your sore throat symptoms suddenly cause a change in your normal voice to what I call a "hot potato" voice. This muffled tone sounds as if you have hot french fries in your mouth and can't fully enunciate. This usually indicates that an abscess has formed in the throat and pus is collecting beyond the wall of the tonsils. Both the throat and tongue may swell when this happens. Other symptoms include a fever of 103 degrees F; swollen, tender glands in the neck; and difficulty in swallowing.

Also contact your doctor if your sore throat persists for more than three days. This is usually a symptom of a bacteria-related problem. Also, if you have an accompanying earache, call your doctor. A sore throat can cause the earache by stimulating Jacobson's nerve, the nerve fibers that go into both the ear and throat.

What the Doctor Will Do

After taking a medical history, if a doctor sees pus on the throat, he will take a throat culture with a special cotton-tipped swab. To get a good sample the doctor will dig deep into the folds of the tonsils, which may cause some discomfort, but the more material he can get on the swab, the more accurate his diagnosis will be. If pus is found, antibiotics such as penicillin or erythromycin will be prescribed.

If a child has three or more strep throats a year, or more than five non-strep sore throats a year that require doctor vis-its, or if the tonsils enlarge so that they interfere with the child's breathing at night, then a tonsillectomy may be in order. In these cases, instead of fighting off infection, the tonsils are acting as sources of infection and should be removed. This won't eliminate sore throats, but will reduce their frequency.

It's not uncommon for adults to have tonsillitis. If recurrent sore throats interfere with your life, then a tonsillectomy may be in order. If you opt for surgery, you will trade one week of throat pain after the tonsillectomy for a greatly reduced number of sore throats.

WHAT TO DO

- Suck on a throat lozenge or a hard candy throughout the day.
- Gargle throughout the day with a mixture of a teaspoonful of salt stirred into 8 ounces of warm water.
- Use a humidifier or a cool-mist vaporizer in your bedroom at night to add extra moisture to the air.
- Take 2 aspirin, acetaminophen, or ibuprofen tablets every four hours to relieve throat pain and inflammation. (Children should not take aspirin because of the danger of Reye's syndrome.)
- Contact a doctor immediately if, in addition to the sore throat, your voice develops a muffled sound, if your tongue and throat swell, and fever goes to 103 degrees F. Also, contact your doctor if the sore throat lasts longer than three days, or you develop an earache.

Strictly Women

GENERAL INFORMATION

Women have special health concerns specifically related to their reproductive organs. Inflammations and infections can affect the cervix, uterus, ovaries, vagina, and vulva, while the reproductive cycle itself can occasionally cause discomfort and anxiety.

A basic understanding of your own body combined with self-help measures described in this section may help you recog-

continued on page 133

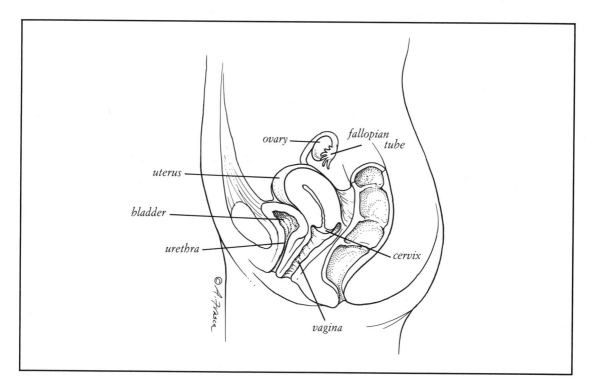

COMMON FEMALE PROBLEMS

MENSTRUAL CRAMPS
Cramps appear on or before menstruation, and are typified by painful intermittent contractions of the uterus. They are sometimes accompanied by backache, nausea, and vomiting.   **Page 134**

PMS
Premenstrual syndrome is a group of distressing symptoms ranging from mild to severe that occurs mainly in the last half of the menstrual cycle, but in some women may develop earlier in the menstrual cycle.   **Page 135**

VAGINITIS
This infection or irritation of the vagina has symptoms that include vaginal itching, discharge, and odor that can range from mild to severe.   **Page 137**

URINARY STRESS INCONTINENCE
The uncontrollable leaking of urine is usually caused by a weakening of the pelvic floor muscles due to pregnancy, obesity, injury, or aging.   **Page 140**

nize and treat various ailments. When a condition appears to be severe at the outset or when the self-help measures don't immediately bring relief, contact your doctor.

FEMALE HEALTH CARE SPECIALISTS

GYNECOLOGIST (M.D.). A gynecologist is a medical doctor who specializes in diagnosing and treating disorders and diseases affecting a woman's reproductive organs. The doctor performs surgery when necessary. Many gynecologists also handle obstetrics.

OBSTETRICIAN (M.D.). An obstetrician specializes in prenatal care, childbirth, and postpartum follow-up.

PHYSICIAN'S CARE REQUIRED

AMENORRHEA. Absence of menstrual periods may be caused by hypothalamus and hormone disorders, depression, diabetes, anorexia nervosa, vigorous exercise, extreme weight loss, medication, or oral contraceptives. If you are not pregnant but have missed periods for six months, contact your physician for an examination.

DYSMENORRHEA. Painful or difficult menstruation characterized by abdominal cramping and pain in the lower back. May signal underlying disorder. Doctor will examine and treat.

FIBROIDS. Benign, slow-growing uterine tumors ranging from minuscule to grapefruit size, which generally disappear after menopause. If you are bothered by heavy menstrual periods or abdominal tenderness, you should be examined regularly. Surgery may be recommended.

LUMP IN BREAST. Most breast lumps are uncomfortable and tender, and all are cause for concern. However, breast lumps are not usually malignant. They are typically caused by a cyst, benign growth, infection, thickening of milk-producing glands, or injury. If a lump develops, consult your doctor, and if necessary, seek the recommended procedures for lump removal.

SEXUALLY TRANSMITTED DISEASES. There are a number of STDs, and they appear to be on the increase. The major risk factor is unprotected sex with an infected partner. Many STDs, such as gonorrhea and HIV, remain symptomless for months or years. Even syphilis may take one to three months before a telltale ulcerous sore appears in the genital area. If you have *any* reason to suspect you may have an STD, consult your physician.

URINARY TRACT INFECTIONS. A bacterial infection caused by incomplete drainage of the bladder and urinary tract, constipation, pregnancy, or irritation and swelling of the urethra following the onset of initial sexual activity, and after resumption of sexual intercourse following a period of abstinence. Painful, foul-smelling, "burning," and frequent urinations are typical symptoms. Cystitis, the most common urinary tract infection, is confined to the bladder. Fever, nausea, and back pain are symptoms of acute pyelonephritis, a kidney infection caused by a urinary tract infection that moved from the bladder to the kidneys. Contact your physician for diagnosis and antibiotic treatment.

MENSTRUAL CRAMPS

Johanna F. Perlmutter, M.D.

Dr. Perlmutter is assistant professor of Obstetrics–Gynecology at Harvard Medical School; obstetrician/gynecologist at Beth Israel Hospital in Boston, Massachusetts

For many women, menstrual cramps and the discomfort they cause are typified not only by cramping of the uterus, but also by stomach and back pain or pain that shoots down the legs. The cramps may be accompanied by nausea and vomiting.

Cramping is generally caused in a healthy woman by the normal release of prostaglandins in the uterus at the time of menstruation. These hormonelike substances cause the uterus to contract, which then leads to the painful cramps.

Treatment

For relief of painful menstrual cramps and their associated discomfort, start with a hot bath. The water helps relax the uterus and any other tensions that may be contributing to the problem.

Place a hot water bottle or a heating pad on your abdomen. The flow of heat can provide soothing, temporary pain relief.

Take acetaminophen tablets for cramp relief by following the dosage recommendations on the container. If you don't feel better, switch to ibuprofen.

Most menstrual cramp pains can be relieved by taking prostaglandin-inhibiting medications now available OTC. Ibuprofen medication (Advil and Motrin), mefenamic acid (Ponstel), and naproxen (Naprosyn) work quite well. Dosage levels depend on the severity of your symptoms. Some women can take 1 tablet every four hours for adequate relief, especially if this is done at the first sign of pain. Others may have to take higher dosages. Notify your physician if you feel it necessary to exceed the dose recommendations on the package.

A traditional way of treating cramping pain prior to prostaglandin inhibitors was alcohol. Alcohol is a good uterine relaxant, and a shot of hard liquor such as whiskey, bourbon, or scotch works well. This is not to recommend use or excessive use of alcohol. As with any other drug, alcohol should be taken with caution.

Exercise regularly. Aerobic exercise such as walking, swimming, running, bicycling, and aerobic dance may diminish cramping symptoms. For some women, exercise may inhibit prostaglandins or help release endorphins, the brain's natural painkillers.

Cause for Concern

If you still fail to get appreciable relief after trying these varied remedies, or if you experience painful cramping that lasts longer than three days, or cramping appears in between your periods, see your gynecologist to make sure that you don't have any underlying problems.

What the Doctor Will Do

After taking a careful history and performing a physical exam, the doctor may prescribe more potent antiprostaglandin medication, or oral contraceptives, which have been known to reduce the painful cramps.

When pain is severe and not controllable with these methods, a laparoscopy—in which the doctor looks inside the peritoneal cavity with a special instrument—may be performed in order to examine the pelvic organs.

WHAT TO DO

- Exercise regularly.
- Take a hot bath.
- Place a hot water bottle or heating pad on your abdomen.
- Take acetaminophen tablets. Follow the dosage recommendations on the container.
- Take OTC prostaglandin-inhibiting medications if acetaminophen doesn't work.
- Contact your gynecologist if you still fail to get appreciable relief after trying these varied remedies, if you experience painful cramping that lasts longer than three days, or if cramping appears between your periods.

PMS

Sally K. Severino, M.D.

Dr. Severino is associate professor of Psychiatry at New York Hospital–Cornell Medical Center in White Plains, New York

Premenstrual syndrome, more commonly known as PMS, includes a range of symptoms from minor to incapacitating. For most women, the symptoms arise shortly before menstruation, but in severe cases they start at the time of ovulation and continue to the onset of bleeding.

There are now over 150 symptoms linked to PMS—the most common include nervous tension, mood swings, irritability, depression, fatigue, headache, insomnia, craving for sweets and salt, abdominal bloating, swelling of the breasts, breast tenderness, and difficulty concentrating. Severe cases seriously disrupt the lives of 3 to 5 percent of women each month.

Although an estimated 10–15 million American women experience premenstrual symptoms to some degree each month, only a small percentage seek treatment for them. They either think there is no solution, or they can't find a doctor to help them. Even with all the PMS research, its cause is still not understood, and doctors are at a loss for a single treatment to eliminate it. Currently, the best treatment for mild to moderate PMS is to manage individual symptoms as they occur.

Treatment

A good strategy to combat PMS symptoms is to keep a detailed diary. Note when symptoms occur, what they include, and how intense they are. Check your diary over a period of months to identify troublesome symptoms. This will help you understand how they are linked to PMS. You can then take actions to alleviate these symptoms.

Water retention is often a major symptom of PMS. Except for severe cases where women actually gain weight from it, I don't recommend diuretics because they can have a negative effect on the body's delicate balance of potassium and sodium electrolytes. (Diuretics are prescription drugs that help increase the elimination of bodily fluids through urination.)

Instead of diuretics, restrict salt intake a few days before your period. This may reduce bloating and any temporary weight gain. If you don't add salt to your food, read food labels to make sure you are not eating a high-sodium diet.

To reduce food cravings, change your diet during the premenstrual period, adding more complex carbohydrates such as vegetables, fruits, pasta, and rice and other grains.

Eat more evenly spaced meals. For example, if you plan to eat a sandwich for lunch, have half of it at midmorning, the other half at regular lunchtime, followed up by a snack at midafternoon.

Eliminate caffeinated products such as soft drinks, chocolate, coffee, and tea from your diet just prior to your period. This can help cut down on irritability, anxiety, and insomnia.

Alcoholic beverages may or may not have an adverse effect on PMS. Some women find their depression intensified by a drink, while others are not bothered at all. Women should be aware that they may be more sensitive to alcohol when they are premenstrual.

OTC pills, powders, and potions for PMS are to be used with caution. Scientific evidence has not proved that vitamins can cure PMS, including vitamins B_6 and E.

Exercise can have a positive effect on mood and sense of well-being. Exercise also seems to give a woman time to herself away from chronic stress. As long as the exercise isn't another way of adding a burden to her already overburdened schedule, it may be recommended. Although exercise may not eliminate all PMS symptoms, it should certainly help promote good health habits.

What the Doctor Will Do

If you think that you have PMS and these self-help measures don't work, contact a doctor. Make sure the doctor believes there is a medical condition called PMS and is willing to put in the time for an extensive evaluation of your case. Also, it's important to make certain your symptoms are due to PMS, and not caused by other conditions such as anemia, thyroid disease, diabetes, or a mood disorder.

For doctor referrals in your area, contact a local medical school and ask for the names of doctors who provide PMS treatment.

As a rule, after several months of doctor-prescribed exercise, diet modification, implementation of stress-management techniques, and self-rating to establish the degree of PMS symptom severity, improvement is felt. However, in some cases, antidepressant medication may be prescribed by the doctor as a last resort to relieve the extremes of depression associated with PMS.

WHAT TO DO

- Keep a diary to note when symptoms occur and what they are.

- Restrict salt intake to help reduce bloating symptoms and weight gain from water retention.
- Change your diet during the premenstrual period. Emphasize more complex carbohydrates and more evenly spaced meals to reduce food cravings.
- Eliminate caffeinated foods to help reduce irritability, anxiety, and insomnia.
- Abstain from alcohol.
- Take ibuprofen or other OTC pain relievers if bothered by premenstrual headaches.
- Use OTC pills, powders, and potions for PMS with caution.
- Exercise regularly.
- If you think that you have PMS and these measures don't lessen your symptoms, contact a doctor who treats PMS.

VAGINITIS

Michael S. Burnhill, M.D., D.M. Sc.

Dr. Burnhill is professor of Clinical Obstetrics and Gynecology at the Robert Wood Johnson Medical School in New Brunswick, New Jersey

Vaginitis is a common infection of the vagina that affects upward of 10 million women of all ages each year. Symptoms appear in the vulvovaginal area, and include itching, discharge, burning sensation, and foul odor.

It's normal to have a slight discharge from the vagina. Healthy women may also smell of perspiration and have a vaguely musky odor, particularly after menstruation, but the odor should never be unpleasant or "fishy." Odors are generally caused by a yeast infection, by the trichomonad parasite, or by bacteria.

Yeast Infection
A yeast infection may be triggered by a high sugar diet, poor control of diabetes, decreased immunity, lack of sleep, hormonal changes due to pregnancy, oral contraceptives, antibiotics, and corticosteroids. Some drugs destroy protective bac-

teria in the intestine and vagina, replacing them with more harmful bacteria and yeast, typically the *Candida albicans* organism.

Symptoms include itching, redness, discomfort, and possibly a cheesy white discharge. This infection can be transmitted to a sexual partner and needs prompt attention.

Treatment

If the infection is linked with the use of antibiotics, you have to restore the basic balance of microorganisms in your intestines and vagina. Purchase a form of harmless bacteria such as lactobacillus or acidophilus in either powder or capsule form at your local health food store. These bacteria are considered "friendly" organisms in the intestines. Make sure the brand has at least 1–2 *billion* organisms per gram. Take according to directions, generally not with meals.

Two former prescription-only medications now available OTC are clotrimazole and miconazole. They are ingredients in such products as Gyne-Lotrimin and Monistat. An applicator full of cream once or twice a day for a week is recommended. If symptoms persist, medical care is indicated.

Douching is a simple and inexpensive way to reduce recurrences of yeast vaginitis. Dissolve 1 tablespoon of boric acid in 1 quart of warm, distilled water. Make sure your syringe is cleaned and rinsed before use. If you are using a disposable unit, discard after one use. Mix according to directions. Sit on the toilet bowl, insert the syringe into the vagina, and raise the bag 2 feet above your hips. When you are fin-

ished, clean the equipment thoroughly or dispose of it.

Trichomoniasis

Infection caused by the trichomonad parasite can be caused by sexual intercourse with an infected partner. Symptoms include an odorous discharge—frothy, green-yellow, and unpleasant—plus internal itching and burning.

Treatment

There is no effective home remedy, although a salt-water douche may provide *temporary* relief. To prepare your salt water solution, dissolve 1 heaping tablespoon of salt in 1 quart of water. In all cases, consult your physician.

Bacterial Vaginitis

Bacterial vaginitis symptoms include itching and a grayish discharge with an odor of fish or ammonia. In some cases, bacterial vaginitis may be triggered by a foreign body, such as a tampon or contraceptive diaphragm.

Treatment

For symptomatic relief, mix 1 ounce of hydrogen peroxide in 1 pint of distilled water and apply with an irrigator.

Prevention

If you have no vaginal discharge, but vaginal itching and burning, try some of the following preventive measures:

- Wash the genital area daily. Use a *hypoallergenic* soap. Chemicals used in many scented deodorant soaps will irritate the vagina. *Be sure to wash all residual soap away carefully.*
- Avoid bubble baths. The chemicals can be irritating.
- After taking a bath, immediately take a shower to make sure that no soap film is left on the body.
- If you take a shower, be sure to rinse off all soap residue from the vulvovaginal area. Dry off after the shower with your own towel.
- Shampoo your hair in the sink and not in the shower where the shampoo can run down and over the pubic area and remain as residual film.
- Use washing detergent that is color- and perfume-free.
- Do not use fabric softeners or chemical bleach.
- Wash all clothing a second time without any detergent to rinse out the remaining soap.
- Use chemical-free, white toilet paper.
- Rinse the vulvovaginal area with warm water after urinating and moving your bowels. Wipe yourself from the front of the anus to the back to avoid introducing new bacteria to the vagina.
- Trapped moisture is one of the primary causes of vaginitis. Keep perspiration to a minimum by wearing cotton underwear or underwear with a cotton crotch. Change daily.
- Instead of pantyhose, wear thigh-high stockings or regular stockings with a garter belt. If you must wear pantyhose, use the type with an absorbent cotton crotch, or else cut out the crotch area.
- Don't sleep in your underwear. Wear a nightgown or loose pajamas.

- Wear jeans or pants that are loose fitting in the crotch and thigh area.
- Only wear exercise clothing that will absorb perspiration. Get out of sweaty gym clothing and wet bathing suits as quickly as possible. Rinse the vulvovaginal area with warm water.
- When urination burns from an irritated vulvovaginal area, moisten the area with a chemical-free and preservative-free vegetable oil or vitamin E oil to protect it from sweat and urine.
- When you urinate, separate the vaginal lips with your fingers. Immediately after urination, rinse with cool water so you don't leave any urine in or around the irritated tissue.
- Make sure your sex partner has washed his genitals before intercourse. Use a condom for added protection.
- Avoid anal intercourse.
- Avoid using tampons until vaginitis is over. After that, use brands made of pure cotton and change frequently during the day.
- For recurrent vaginitis, avoid tampons for three to four months because of their tendency to increase undesirable organisms in the vagina. Instead, buy a roll of absorbent cotton, tear off pieces, and use them for spotting or discharge.
- Don't use any powder in the vaginal area. It tends to be an irritant.

Cause for Concern

If you don't get relief in a few days, or if your symptoms worsen, go to a knowledgeable professional trained to identify and treat vaginitis. This can be a nurse clinician or a physician's assistant, as well as a gynecologist or family practitioner. It is practically impossible to diagnose vaginitis correctly over the telephone or merely by looking at it.

What the Doctor Will Do

Every case requires the doctor to figure out if the vaginitis comes from a sex partner, a chemical sensitivity, or an infection, or if an underlying intestinal or medical disorder is the primary cause.

- A detailed medical history will be taken.
- The discharge will be cultured and examined with a microscope to make a correct diagnosis.
- Medication will be provided when the personal history, physical examination, and laboratory study have led to an appropriate diagnosis.

WHAT TO DO

- Take bacteria such as acidophilus in dosages of 1 to 2 billion organisms per gram if your condition is caused by the use of antibiotics.

- Use baking soda solution douche.

If you have no vaginal discharge, but itching and burning in the vagina:

- Avoid all deodorant or perfumed soaps.
- Wash the genital area daily with a hypoallergenic soap to be sure all residual soap is rinsed away.
- Immediately rinse in the shower after taking a bath to wash off residual soap.
- Shampoo your hair in the sink to avoid leaving shampoo or hair conditioner in the vulvovaginal area.
- Wash all clothing a second time without any detergent. Avoid bleach, fabric softener, perfumes, and coloring agents.
- Air-dry undergarments.
- Use white, unscented toilet paper.
- Wear cotton underwear or underwear with a cotton crotch.
- Use only exercise clothing with an absorbent crotch.
- Make sure your sex partner washes his genitals before intercourse.
- If you've observed all these precautions and don't see relief in three days, or if symptoms worsen, contact a knowledgeable clinician.

URINARY STRESS INCONTINENCE

José Sotolongo, M.D.

Dr. Sotolongo is associate professor of Urology at Mount Sinai Medical School and attending urologist at the Mount Sinai Incontinence Clinic in New York City

For many women with urinary stress incontinence, everyday activities such as playing sports, lifting up the baby, coughing, sneezing, and even laughing can trigger involuntary urination.

A woman may lose anywhere from a

few drops of urine to up to a half cup several times a day. The disorder is vastly underreported, and possibly 10 percent of all women have it.

Urinary stress incontinence is often inherited—the woman is born with a urethra, the tube that leads out of the bladder, that is too short. Many times the incontinence is related to the weakening of the pelvic floor muscles caused by childbirth or obesity. These muscles, which are responsible for holding up the vagina, bladder, and urethra, are sometimes stretched and lose their strength, and thus the ability of the urinary sphincter to hold urine in the bladder is diminished. When this happens, any subsequent increase of abdominal pressure on the bladder from straining or jumping brings on an embarrassing leak.

Treatment

If stress incontinence is linked to obesity, the problem may be resolved over time through weight loss. Combining dietary restriction and regular exercise is the safest and most effective way to lose weight; crash diets don't work in the long run.

When the degree of incontinence is slight, Kegel exercise, which helps strengthen the pubococcygeal muscles that affect bladder control, may also be helpful.

To perform the Kegel exercise, contract your anal sphincter as you would to prevent a bowel movement. Hold for a few seconds and then relax. Repeat this exercise thirty times, three times daily.

What the Doctor Will Do

If weight loss and special exercises fail to eliminate the problem, contact your physician.

- After an exam, antibiotics will be prescribed if a urinary infection is contributing to or causing your problems.
- If you don't have an infection, a surgical procedure called a urethral suspension may be performed to bring the bladder and urethra back up into the abdomen. Typically, two days of hospitalization are required, and the operation has a 95 percent success rate.

If your incontinence is slight, or if you choose not to have the surgery, you can opt for wearing a minipad to absorb urine and to prevent odor and chafing. As a temporary solution, this may be helpful, but in general, minipads are not recommended for long-term treatment.

WHAT TO DO

- Lose weight with diet and exercise if the problem is linked with obesity.
- Perform Kegel exercise twice daily to help strengthen the muscles that affect bladder control.
- If weight loss and the special exercise fails to eliminate urinary stress incontinence, contact your family physician to check for a urinary infection. In some cases surgery is an option.

The Feet

GENERAL INFORMATION

The twenty-six bones of each foot are held in place by tendons, ligaments, and muscles that bend, twist, and flex so we can walk, run, and jump. With every footstep, a force two to three times the weight of the body comes down on the foot, and this increased force is almost tripled when we are running or jumping. The sole of the foot is thickly padded with fat and a dense layer of skin to help buffer these stresses.

When the feet function properly, the

continued on page 144

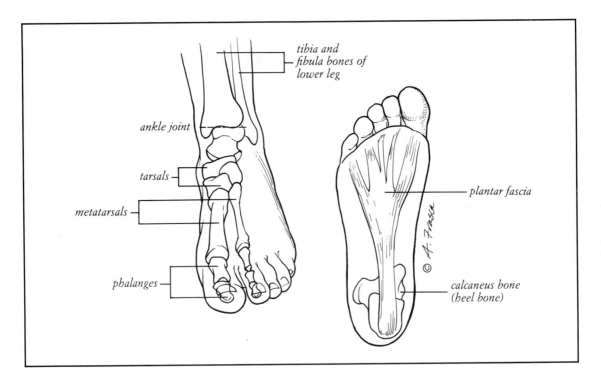

tibia and
fibula bones of
lower leg

ankle joint

tarsals

metatarsals

phalanges

plantar fascia

calcaneus bone
(heel bone)

© A. Frasca

COMMON FOOT PROBLEMS

ATHLETE'S FOOT
When feet are kept warm and moist, this sometimes painful and chronic fungal infection thrives. Symptoms include itchy, scaly, oozing, and reddened skin; patches between the toes; and scaling along the sides and soles of the feet. Athlete's foot can affect and destroy toenails. **Page 144**

BUNION
This unsightly and painful deformity of the big toe joint is aggravated by ill-fitting shoes but not caused by them. Temporary measures offer some relief, but surgery is often required. **Page 146**

CORNS AND CALLUSES
Excessive pressure against the bony areas of the feet causes corns, which are compacted dead skin cells. Hard corns typically appear on the tops of the toes and soft corns appear between the toes. Calluses are rough, thickened areas of yellowish skin that form over prominent bone structures to protect those areas from being irritated by poorly fitting shoes, friction, and heat buildup. Calluses themselves can become painful. They are typically found on the toes, the heel, the ball of the foot, or on the side of the big toe joint. **Page 147**

FOOT ODOR
This condition often results from excessive perspiration that provides an environment for bacteria. **Page 150**

HEEL AND ARCH PAIN
Plantar fasciitis, an aggravation of the tough fibrous band that runs from the heel to the ball of the foot, is the most common cause. This dull ache feels worse in the morning and eases with continual movement. A long recovery period is needed for moderate to severe cases. **Page 151**

INGROWN TOENAIL
This painful condition can result from a number of systemic diseases, ill-fitting shoes, improperly trimmed toenails, or injury. Infection is common. **Page 154**

SORE FEET
A common problem after extensive walking, running, and jumping, most often caused by improper footwear. **Page 156**

rest of the kinetic chain—the knees, hips, spine, and neck—usually function well. However, something as innocuous as a foot splinter can upset the biomechanics of the kinetic chain and may lead to disabling stresses to the body's musculoskeletal system.

Daily hygiene that includes washing and drying the feet is important to ward off bacteria and fungus. Proper footwear is also imperative. Ill-fitting shoes are a cause of many foot ailments.

FOOT CARE SPECIALISTS

ORTHOPEDIST (M.D.). An orthopedist is a medical doctor who specializes in the diagnosis, treatment, and prevention of disorders to the musculoskeletal system, including bones, joints, ligaments, tendons, muscles, and nerves. An orthopedist performs surgery when necessary.

OSTEOPATH (D.O.). An osteopath is a trained specialist who can prescribe medication and also do massage, physical manipulation, and rehabilitation techniques to enhance recovery from injury or disease. Osteopaths are not medical doctors.

PHYSICAL THERAPIST (P.T.). A registered physical therapist is trained to provide techniques and services for aiding recovery and restoring proper movement to the body. In many states, a doctor's prescription is needed for treatment by a physical therapist.

PODIATRIST (D.P.M.). A podiatrist specializes in the diagnosis, treatment, and prevention of foot disorders resulting from injury or disease. A D.P.M. makes independent judgments, prescribes medications, and performs surgery when necessary. Podiatrists are not medical doctors.

ATHLETE'S FOOT

Rodney S. W. Basler, M.D.

Dr. Basler is chairman of the Sportsmedicine Task Force for the American Academy of Dermatology, and an assistant professor of Internal Medicine at the University of Nebraska Medical Center in Omaha

Athlete's foot, or tinea pedis, is a common, generally harmless foot infection caused by fungi that thrive in warm, moist, and dark environments. Wearing poorly ventilated shoes and socks that don't wick away perspiration provide an ideal breeding ground for these germs that quickly multiply to cause athlete's foot.

Typical symptoms include scaling and peeling in the toe webs (the area between the toes) generally without any accompanying pain, odor, or itching. Some forms of athlete's foot may present as redness, blistering, and scaling along the sides and soles of the feet, taking on what's termed a moccasin pattern. In more advanced cases, the toe webs develop whitened, softened, soggy skin; severe itching; and some odor. As the condition worsens, painful cracking in the toe webs and some oozing may develop. If it stays long enough, athlete's foot will eventually affect the toenails, developing a crumbly white texture, and causing the nails to thicken. In advanced cases this can become very painful.

If you don't have the proper immunity, I think you're destined to a lifetime of athlete's foot. I've had it since I was fifteen years old and have been battling it constantly ever since.

Treatment

Treatment for athlete's foot is simple, uncomplicated, and carried out at home. When it first appears, I go to my medicine cabinet and take out the clotrimazole (brand names: Mycelex or Lotrimin) lotion. This former prescription-only item is now available OTC in cream and lotion form and is effective in knocking out the fungus.

Here's a trick to treatment: twice daily use the clotrimazole cream on the soles of your feet and also in the groin area if you have jock itch (see JOCK ITCH, page 195), an ailment often caused by the same fungi as athlete's foot. But for your toe webs, it's important that you only use clotrimazole *lotion* because it will be quickly absorbed and won't trap moisture, as the cream will. This moisture could eventually prolong the problem by softening the skin.

When I treat my athlete's foot for three consecutive days immediately after noticing symptoms, it disappears for at least ninety days. However, if you're lazy about treatment, or delay treatment, it can quickly become painful, and you will need to see a dermatologist.

Prevention

Athlete's foot is stubborn and will return when the conditions are right, no matter what commonsense precautions you may take. To delay or help prevent its onset, carry out the following procedures after bathing and swimming:

- Always dry your feet, paying particular attention to the toe webs. Athlete's foot is slightly contagious, so don't use the same towel or bathmat as other family members.
- After drying, apply antifungal lotion and follow this with an antifungal foot powder. Zeasorb AF is good because it contains no cornstarch, a substance that can encourage fungal growth.
- Wear socks made of absorbent fibers like cotton, and change them daily.
- When your feet are going to perspire excessively for extended periods of time, wear socks made of high turbo acrylic fiber. These will wick the moisture away from your feet and carry it to the sock's outer layer to evaporate.
- When the weather is hot and humid, go barefoot whenever possible.
- Avoid tight, poorly ventilated shoes. Sandals or perforated shoes are best.
- Be sure to air your shoes at night and, if possible, don't wear the same street shoes or athletic footwear every day.

What the Doctor Will Do

To make a definitive diagnosis, a doctor will scrape the skin with a surgical blade and study the skin fragments under a microscope. However, in most cases, the doctor will simply examine your feet, determine that it is athlete's foot, and prescribe oral antifungal medication that is taken daily for at least a month. He may also prescribe cream or lotion to apply during this time.

For people with chronic, severe athlete's foot, who are especially miserable and disabled by it in the summer months, I start them on a course of prescription oral medication and prescription lotion in mid-May that they will use until mid-September. This should take care of their major foot symptoms and allow them to enjoy all of their summer activities.

If your toenails begin to thicken so much that they become painful, or if you're bothered by the nails for cosmetic concerns, there is a prescription medication that can be taken for an eighteen-month period, after which the pain will disappear, and the nails will regain their normal texture.

WHAT TO DO

- Dry your feet after bathing, especially between the toes.
- Twice daily, apply clotrimazole lotion to the toe webs and clotrimazole cream to other affected foot parts.
- Wear socks made of absorbent fibers and change them daily.
- Air your shoes at night and, if possible, wear a different pair on alternate days.
- Contact a dermatologist if these steps fail to bring relief.

BUNIONS

Michael J. Trepal, D.P.M.

Dr. Trepal is professor and chairman, Division of Surgical Sciences,
New York College of Podiatric Medicine in New York City

A bunion is a slowly progressing congenital or hereditary ailment that causes the big toe to fall out of alignment with, and drift toward, the second and third toes. As this happens, the ball of the foot directly beneath the big toe becomes more prominent and painful. Encountering friction with the side of the shoe, this area in turn becomes more irritated and swollen. A callus may develop on the overlying skin, and swelling increases and spreads to the big toe joint. It's not uncommon to develop bursitis, a joint inflammation, under the toe joint.

Bunions as a rule affect women more than men, often run in families, and typically become most problematic as a person reaches middle age.

Constricting shoes, high heels, pointed shoes, and tight stockings or socks don't cause bunions, but they can aggravate them. In some advanced bunion cases, the toe may become arthritic. This may lead to stresses on the ankles, knees, hips, and back from walking with an abnormal gait, which can lead to arthritis in those areas as well.

Treatment

If you have a bunion that has become troublesome, avoid shoes with a narrow toe box (the front area of the shoe), and wear lower heels instead of high heels whenever possible.

To keep the pressure off a bunion, you may want to cut a hole or slit in your shoe near the bunion and wear this shoe until the pain has diminished.

Bunion pads are available OTC in the pharmacy. These aids won't cure the bunion, but when applied to the toe, they can bring relief by decreasing the painful friction between shoe and toe.

What the Doctor Will Do

If you have a bunion and can no longer stand the pain, contact a physician who has experience in surgery of the foot. This can be either a podiatrist or an orthopedist.

After confirming you have a bunion, the doctor may alleviate the pain with an injection of cortisone to decrease the swelling in and around the joint. Physical therapy and oral anti-inflammatory medication may also be prescribed, and special padding provided for inside your shoes. All of these measures are palliative. For severe bunions, surgery is recommended. This entails straightening and repositioning the big toe. In this case, a cast is often applied, and it generally takes two months until normal activities can be resumed.

WHAT TO DO

- Do not wear constricting, pointed, or high-heeled shoes.
- Wear shoes with a wide toe box.
- When the toe is especially inflamed and painful, cut a hole near the bunion in a shoe to provide extra room.
- To decrease friction between the shoe and the bunion, apply a bunion pad to the toe.
- If the pain becomes too severe or normal walking is disturbed, contact a podiatrist or an orthopedist who specializes in the feet to obtain an examination.

CORNS AND CALLUSES

Suzanne M. Levine, D.P.M.

Dr. Levine is adjunct clinical professor of Podiatrics at the New York College of Podiatric Medicine in New York City

The skin of the foot reacts to excessive chafing and pressure of ill-fitting shoes by developing corns and calluses.

These are very common foot problems characterized by abnormally thickened layers of dead skin that form over bony areas of the feet. Women tend to have these problems more than men because of changes in weight during pregnancy and the practice of wearing high-heeled shoes.

Corns

There are two types of corns. A hard corn is a painful, rounded, hard layer of skin that develops on the feet and toes, typically over a toe joint. A hard corn first appears as red and then turns yellowish. Direct pressure on this area causes a dull, often penetrating and throbbing pain.

Soft corns usually develop between the fourth and fifth toes either from pressure of these two toes pressing against each other or from excessive moisture in the fourth toe web. A soft corn is often white and painful and sometimes accompanied by athlete's foot (see ATHLETE'S FOOT, page 144).

Prevention

Corns are caused by ill-fitting shoes.

- Wear shoes that fit properly in the toe box.
- Avoid high heels, which push the toes downward into the toe box.
- Discard all ill-fitting shoes. There is no way that you will ever "break them in."

Treatment

The pain associated with corns can be decreased when you reduce the corn or totally eliminate it. There are several ways to remove a corn, but in my mind, only one safe and effective way.

I have developed a four-step method of corn removal that is safe, effective, and easy to do. First, add 3 tablespoons of Epsom salts to a container of warm water large enough to hold your feet. Soak your feet in this mixture for 15 minutes. This will help soften the skin and reduce inflammation caused by the corns.

Dry the feet and apply a layer of your favorite moisturizing cream or petroleum jelly onto the toes with corns. The cream will penetrate and help soften the skin even more. Apply plastic wrap over the affected toes, or wrap the entire foot in a plastic bag, and keep them wrapped for 15 minutes. The ensuing buildup of body heat will make the corn more susceptible to the benefit of a pumice stone.

Do not use a razor to remove a corn. This often leads to damage of the surrounding skin. With a pumice stone, available in any pharmacy, rub the corn gently back and forth to scrape away the hard outer layer of skin, being careful not to abrade the surrounding skin. When finished, apply more moisturizing cream to soothe the area.

Repeat this procedure twice a week until the corn is gone.

To remove a soft corn between the fourth and fifth toes, dry the area completely with a towel after regular bathing, and apply a light dusting of talcum powder or cornstarch. If you have accompanying athlete's foot, apply an antifungal agent (see ATHLETE'S FOOT, page 144).

Always try to keep the feet dry and avoid tight shoes. Wider shoes will relieve the pressure on the fourth and fifth toes, and the soft corn should disappear on its own in two weeks.

I'm not a fan of the over-the-counter medicated corn pad. They are very caustic and can harm healthy skin. Also, people who are diabetic or have vascular problems are at risk if they use these products because serious infection can develop.

Callus

A callus is a rough, thickened piece of yellowish skin that develops after repeated irritation or chafing to any part of the body.

A callus is usually painless, but if it increases in size, it can press on nerve endings and cause discomfort. On the foot, calluses are typically found on the ball, heel, and side, or over a bunion (see BUNION, page 146).

Calluses are caused by ill-fitting shoes or by shoes ill-equipped to handle the pressure exerted on the foot during vigorous activity. Calluses also develop when socks are not worn with sport shoes.

Prevention

- To prevent calluses, wear shoes wide enough and sufficiently cushioned to protect the feet.
- Wear socks if you are prone to calluses.
- Whenever possible, avoid activities that place continued pressure on the skin.

Treatment

If a callus becomes unsightly or so large that it presses into the foot and causes pain, this remedy will help the problem. Take 5–6 plain aspirin tablets and crush them into a fine powder. Mix this powder with 1 tablespoonful of water in a small cup.

Soak your foot, or feet, in warm water and Epsom salts for 15 minutes. After drying your feet, apply this mild aspirin paste to the callus and wrap your entire foot in a plastic bag for 10 minutes. The buildup of body heat allows the salicylic acid from the aspirin paste to penetrate the callus.

Take the bag off and gently use a pumice stone to rub away all the callused skin.

WHAT TO DO

- Discard ill-fitting shoes.
- Wear shoes with a wide toe box.
- When bothered by corns, don't wear high heels. Wear pumps or sandals instead.
- Use the safe and effective four-step corn removal treatment.
- Avoid OTC corn removal products.
- To remove soft corns, after washing and drying the feet, apply a light dusting of talcum powder or cornstarch. Wear wider shoes.
- For callus removal, soak feet in Epsom salt mixture for 15 minutes, apply aspirin paste to the callused area, and use a pumice stone to rub away dead skin.

FOOT ODOR

Thomas M. DeLauro, D.P.M.

Dr. DeLauro is executive vice-president for academic and clinical affairs at the New York College of Podiatric Medicine in New York City

For odor to develop, a foot has to sweat excessively. Most people have foot odor at one time or another in their lives, but a persistent problem is usually confined to individuals who perspire heavily.

For the most part, foot odor clears up with regular hygiene. However, if the condition is linked with a person's underlying stress and tension, the foot odor will continue until these problems are corrected.

Some of the causes of foot sweating include nervous disorders, wearing shoes made of synthetic materials that don't allow normal foot perspiration to evaporate, continuously wearing socks made of synthetic fibers that become damp with perspiration, and wearing the same pair of shoes every day. Even shoes made of the finest leather will not allow perspiration to evaporate completely in twenty-four hours. The damp, dark, and warm environment of the shoe becomes an ideal breeding ground for odor-causing bacteria.

Treatment

Several types of over-the-counter foot powders or sprays are available, but I don't find them to be effective against foot odor. Although it may sound strange, the simplest and most effective treatment is soaking your feet in tea. Tea contains tannic acid, a powerful astringent that will dry the foot and keep it from perspiring.

Patients with diabetes or other disorders that affect circulation should not use this as a treatment without consulting their doctor.

To make a tea-leaf soak, boil water and place it in a pot or pan large enough to accommodate your feet. Add 2 tea bags per quart of water and let them steep for 10 minutes. Make sure that ordinary tea is used, not decaffeinated or herbal tea.

After the liquid has cooled sufficiently, put your feet in the bath and soak them for 15 minutes. Repeat this soak daily until you notice that your feet are no longer perspiring excessively. This generally takes two or three days.

Daily soaking of the feet should not continue after excessive perspiration has stopped. Continuing the treatment at this point may lead to overdrying of the skin and subsequently to cracking and splitting.

The tea-leaf soak should keep your feet from sweating for four to five days. If your feet start to perspire heavily once again, repeat the daily soaks. I find that one soak is all that's needed in subsequent treatments to keep the feet from sweating.

In addition to soaking your feet, don't wear the same shoes every day. Rotate the shoes that you wear during the week, wearing shoes made of leather as often as possible. Weather permitting, wear pure wool socks to keep the feet warm and dry. Wool socks are best at taking perspiration away from the feet and allowing it to evaporate. In any event, be sure to change your socks daily.

In most cases, good daily foot hygiene

helps prevent foot odor. As part of your bathing routine, be sure to wash your feet with warm, soapy water to kill bacteria.

WHAT TO DO

- Wash the feet with soap and warm water to kill bacteria and remove dirt.

- Wear wool socks to take perspiration away from the feet.
- Wear leather shoes. Rotate the shoes you wear daily.
- Try the tea-leaf soak for 15 minutes a day.
- Address the underlying issues of tension and stress that may be causing excessive perspiration.

HEEL AND ARCH PAIN

Stephen I. Subotnick, D.P.M., M.S.

Dr. Subotnick is a professor of Biomechanics at the California College of Podiatric Medicine, San Francisco, California

Most heel and arch pain stems from plantar fasciitis, an injury that typically develops from either too much activity, unaccustomed activity, poorly cushioned shoes, harsh impact, or vibration from continual walking or running on hard surfaces. This stretches the plantar fascia, the fibrous band of connective tissue that is attached to the heel and runs through the arch to the toes.

Microtears in the plantar fascia lead to soreness, stiffness, inflammation, and pain. The pain is usually felt in the arch of the foot and on the bottom of the heel. It is most painful upon arising in the morning, feels better with continued motion, but worsens again with too much activity. The heel and arch also feel worse in damp weather and on colder days.

The pain caused by plantar fasciitis is barely noticeable at first. People often ignore the first signals of dull ache or intermittent pain. But when the condition is ignored for too long and coupled with continued activity, inflammation and unrelenting soreness often result.

Treatment

The best treatment for the pain of plantar fasciitis is six to eight weeks of modified activity. Although you don't have to stop exercising totally, there has to be a reduction in the frequency and intensity of your walking or running. For competitive athletes, a reduction in running by as much as 80 percent may be necessary.

To maintain your cardiovascular fitness, try cross-training instead, and walk or run every third day. Cross-training means alternating activities that you normally do with other activities such as swimming, water aerobics, and bicycling. These provide effective aerobic workouts and also decrease stress to the foot. As the pain diminishes, you can gradually increase the frequency and intensity of your walking or running.

It is also helpful to stretch the calf muscles and Achilles tendons twice a day by performing the following exercise: Stand 3 feet from a wall, stretch your arms out and place palms flat against the wall. Place your right leg 8–12 inches behind you. Keep this leg straight and both heels firmly on the floor. Lean forward into the wall until you feel the calf muscle stretch. Hold this stretch for 15 seconds. Perform the same stretch on the left leg and repeat the stretches a total of three times for both legs.

For treating mild cases of plantar fasciitis, I prefer using heat instead of cold for pain relief. Fill a basin with body temperature water (100–110 degrees F) and add Epsom salts. Soak the feet for 20 minutes, drying them off immediately after.

However, if the heel or arch feels inflamed or hot to the touch, ice treatment may be better. Soak your foot for 20 minutes in a basin filled with ice and water.

Ice massage is another way to relieve inflammation caused by plantar fasciitis. Freeze several paper cups of water. Apply ice to the sore area of the foot, peeling off sections of the cup as the ice melts. Make slow, circular strokes over the heel and arch for 10–15 minutes.

Contrast therapy—using both ice and heat—is another treatment that may bring relief. Try it if you don't have success with hot or cold treatments. Start with your foot in a warm basin (see above) for 30 seconds to 2 minutes and then immediately put it into a basin of ice for 30 seconds to 2 minutes. Repeat this contrast procedure for 10 minutes, ending with a final ice bath.

Aspirin or ibuprofen can help reduce the pain and inflammation of plantar fasciitis. Take 2 ibuprofen tablets three times daily or 2 aspirin tablets twice daily. Continue as long as the pain lasts, but no longer than seven to ten days.

Taping the foot with 2-inch wide surgical tape can give the foot necessary support and reduce pain. This tape is available at any pharmacy. Start taping at the heel and run strips longitudinally along the sole to the ball of the foot. Anchor this tape by running several strips around the ball and top of the foot.

Apply tape before physical activity or use it for four straight days to support the foot for everyday activities.

Full arch supports or heel supports made of viscoelastic polymer are available in sporting goods stores and pharmacies. They offer good shock absorbency and help reduce pain and inflammation. Place them in all of your shoes until the problem abates.

If these supports don't relieve the pain, consult a podiatrist. The doctor may recommend a pair of custom-made orthoses (appliances to improve function). These devices are made of leather, fiberglass, or plastic, and help relieve discomfort.

Treading on hard surfaces can cause plantar fasciitis, so walk or run on a soft surface such as a rubberized track, chip bark trail, grass, or sand whenever possible.

It's also essential to wear shoes with thick, stable heels and adequate arch support. Women should avoid heels higher than 1 inch because they place too much stress on the arch.

Another cause of heel pain is aging. After the age of forty, or earlier if the person is obese or has rheumatoid arthritis, the shock-absorbing pads of fat in the heels start to thin out naturally, and even limited walking can cause heel pain. Place ready-made heel supports made of viscoelastic polymer in your shoes. If these fail to bring relief after two weeks, contact your podiatrist for custom-made heel supports.

Cause for Concern

If you continue to have persistent heel and arch pain in spite of all these measures, contact a podiatrist or orthopedist.

What the Doctor Will Do

After taking a detailed medical history, X rays and possibly a bone scan may be needed to rule out a stress fracture of the heel. This fracture is a small hairline break in the bone caused by repeated pressure on the foot from your daily activity or sports participation. If there is a fracture, a walking cast is usually applied and worn for several weeks.

Generally, for severe or chronic plantar fasciitis, a custom heel support will be made and physical therapy prescribed three times a week. Another part of the treatment may include the anti-inflammatory medication cortisone, which will be injected into the heel.

When heel or arch pain persists for more than eight months to a year following these conservative measures, surgery is often suggested.

WHAT TO DO

- Reduce the frequency and intensity of your walking and running activities.
- If you are involved in a walking or running program, cross-train by alternating bicycling, water aerobics, or swimming with your normal activity for two out of three days.
- Stretch the calf muscles and Achilles tendons twice daily.
- Apply hot or cold treatments, or both, to the heel and arch.
- Take aspirin or ibuprofen for seven days for reduction of inflammation and pain relief.
- Tape the arch with 2-inch surgical tape.
- Wear shoes with thick rubber heels and adequate arch support. Women should not wear heels higher than 1 inch.
- Place full arch or heel supports made of viscoelastic polymer in your shoes.
- If you continue to experience pain and stiffness after utilizing all of these conservative treatments, contact a podiatrist or an orthopedist who specializes in the foot for a complete examination. There are many treatment options available. Custom orthoses may have to be prescribed.

INGROWN TOENAIL

Rock G. Positano, D.P.M., M.P.H., M.Sc.

*Dr. Positano is co-director of the Foot and Ankle Orthopedic Institute at the
Hospital for Special Surgery in New York City*

An ingrown toenail is one of the most common foot problems, afflicting people of all ages. The large toe is usually the one affected. Typical symptoms include pain and red, swollen skin around the margins of the toenail that is hot to the touch and extremely tender. When infection develops, pus may be visible, and a crust of pus may form over the damaged skin.

An ingrown toenail develops when an unusual amount of pressure is applied to the toe. The edge of the toenail then cuts into the nail bed, the soft tissue surrounding the nail. This leads to pain and often infection, as the nail continues to grow and push into the skin. In extreme cases, the infection may spread from the big toe to other parts of the foot.

There are several causes of ingrown toenails, but wearing ill-fitting shoes is the most common. Shoes should fit comfortably when you try them on, which means they should not rub, pinch, or bind the front of your feet in the area known as the toe box. Many people think they have to "break in" new shoes. This is a mistake that often leads to ingrown toenails.

Another prime cause of ingrown toenails is what I call "bathroom surgery," the often botched attempts at trimming the toenails. Many people cut their toenails along the natural curve of the big toe, which may leave sharp corners of the nail that can grow into the nail fold. The same result can happen when you cut the toenail too short, allowing surrounding tissue to grow over the nail.

Whenever I cut my toenails, I always cut straight across the top of the nail with nail scissors. Using a nail file or emery board, I carefully round off the edges of the nail closest to the nail fold, being careful not to scrape the skin.

Another cause of ingrown toenails are so-called professional pedicures. Many people who trim toenails have no knowledge of nail structure, and trim the nails too short. Often they damage the nail bed by using metal instruments on the nail and cuticle. This practice can lead not only to ingrown toenails, but also to paronychia, a bacterial or fungal infection that must be treated with prescription medication.

A foreign body—such as a grain of sand or a strand of hair—trapped in the nail fold can lead to an ingrown toenail. To avoid this, be wary whenever you walk barefooted or wear sandals. Check your nail beds daily for any foreign matter that may have become trapped, and if you find some foreign matter, ease it out gently with a nail file.

Trauma can also cause an ingrown toenail. If you drop something on your toe or accidentally stub it, the impact may break the nail or force the nail into the nail bed, leading to an ingrown toenail. To avoid this, wear sturdy shoes to protect your feet, especially whenever you perform manual labor.

If your nail has been torn or broken by accident, be sure to use scissors to trim the nail. Never attempt to pull a jagged nail off with your fingers. You risk ripping and tearing deep into the nail bed, which can easily lead to infection.

Treatment

The old wives' tale of cutting a V-shaped wedge out of the middle of your toenail to reduce the inflammation is a fallacy. Instead, get a packet of Domeboro Soaks, available at any pharmacy. Following the mixing instructions, soak your foot each night for 20 minutes to drain out inflamed material under the nail and significantly reduce swelling. Between soaks, apply an antibiotic ointment.

To help the ingrown nail grow over the nail fold, after the nightly soaking, take a tiny bit of cotton and gently wedge it under the ingrown nail. The cotton will act as a buttress and cushion, allowing the skin to be free of excessive nail pressure. Change the cotton every day and continue to use it until the nail has finally grown out past the nail fold.

Cause for Concern

If you suffer increased pain due to an ingrown toenail and it becomes difficult to walk, or if infection of the surrounding skin is accompanied by a fever, contact your physician.

What the Doctor Will Do

A doctor will apply a local anesthetic and then begin to free up the borders of the nail. Using a special instrument called an English anvil, he will slide the instrument under the nail, pushing it straight back to the cuticle. The anvil neatly cuts out that sliver of nail that is growing into the flesh. Once this nail has been removed, all pressure is taken off the toe skin, and relief is almost instantaneous.

The toe is then wrapped in sterile dressing and oral antibiotic medication is prescribed for a ten-day period. Each night the foot is soaked for a half hour in an antibacterial solution mixed in warm water. The healthy nail will be in place in one to two months.

WHAT TO DO

- Wear comfortable shoes with a wide toe box.
- Cut toenails straight across, carefully trimming the sides of the nails with an emery board or nail file.
- Be wary of professional pedicurists.
- If you go barefoot or wear sandals, check the nailfolds for any soil or debris that may have become lodged there.
- Do not use your fingers to rip or pull off a torn or jagged nail.
- If an ingrown toenail occurs, soak your foot nightly in a warm water solution for 20 minutes to reduce inflammation and swelling.
- Apply an antibiotic ointment.
- To help an ingrown toenail grow over the nail fold, gently wedge a piece of cotton under the nail edge after soaking the foot.
- If the pain becomes unbearable, or if it becomes difficult to walk, or if infection has increased and is accompanied by a fever, contact your physician.

SORE FEET

Irwin L. Bliss, M.D.

Dr. Bliss is assistant clinical professor, Department of Orthopedics, UCLA School of Medicine, and medical director, West Los Angeles Foot and Ankle Center

A simple complaint of tired, sore, swollen, or painful feet can mean something totally different for each person. The key to treating sore feet is to find the cause of the discomfort. In some cases, it may not be a foot problem at all.

It's not unusual to experience foot discomfort after walking, running, jumping, or standing on your feet all day. However, many foot problems are linked with the shoes you wear.

High heels are a major source of foot discomfort. The raised heels stress the feet and toes by exerting pressure on the toes and ball of the foot.

Tight shoes, obesity, and repeated foot trauma can also cause neuromas to develop on the sole of the forefoot. A neuroma, a knotting of the nerve fibers that go from the second, third, and fourth toes, causes shooting pains in the forefoot. Jumping, dancing, and trying to run with a neuroma may cause unbearable pain.

Treatment

If you have a neuroma, consult an orthopedist or podiatrist for an evaluation. Conservative treatment is initially advised. In some cases, inserting a small felt pad in the innersole of the shoe, just in front of the tender area, will help relieve pressure.

Another way to alleviate the discomfort of a neuroma is to switch to wider shoes, giving the feet more room to spread out and thereby alleviating pressure on the neuroma.

If you wear athletic shoes with full sole inserts and need to determine the area of the shoe that is pressing on the neuroma, take lipstick and apply it to the spot on your foot where the tenderness is felt. Then put your bare foot into the athletic shoe and walk around the room. Take out the insole of the shoe and you will see a red mark from the lipstick. This is the spot where the shoe is pressing on the neuroma.

Cut a hole through the insole with scissors. Then when you wear your shoe the sole will no longer be pressing against the neuroma. Although this won't make the neroma go away, there should be less pressure on the surrounding tissue, and you should feel less pain.

When the arches of your feet ache after walking around during the day, or if they feel stiff after taking part in vigorous sports activity, it could mean the ligaments supporting your feet are strained.

If you have this problem, purchase a pair of the arch supports sold in pharmacies and athletic shoe stores. Most arch supports are made of sponge rubber or some other shock absorbing material and covered with leather. Slip them into your shoes and wear them for two weeks. If they help, continue to wear them in all of your shoes.

When your feet feel weary at the end of the day, give yourself a foot massage. Add some moisturizer to your sole and gently rub it into the foot with your thumb in a gentle circular motion. Although this massage won't do anything for your circulation, if it feels good, it may be all that you need in order to ease that day's strain on your feet and help you to feel more comfortable.

The "air alphabet" is an excellent exercise to stretch out your foot and ankle and make them feel relaxed. The best position for writing the alphabet is sitting down in a high chair so your feet are hanging free. Starting with your right foot, pretend that your big toe is holding a pen. Begin to write out the twenty-six letters of the alphabet in the air with your foot. Focus your movements on your foot and try not to move your leg. After completing the alphabet, you will have moved every joint in your foot and ankle. Repeat the process with the left foot.

Whenever your feet are swollen at the end of the day, *and if you don't have any vascular problems,* lie down and prop your feet up on some pillows so they are higher than the level of your heart. This will help drain the fluid out of the feet and make you feel more comfortable.

If a vascular problem with your legs and feet has been diagnosed, elevating your feet above your heart may complicate blood flow. Instead, to get some relief from the swelling and discomfort, lie down but keep the feet *at heart level.*

Don't smoke. Smoking cigarettes is terrible for the feet. As you smoke, blood vessels are constricted and blood flow to the feet is reduced by as much as 50 percent. Anyone with a preexisting circulation problem in the feet or legs does himself or herself great harm by smoking.

Plunge your tired, aching feet into a cold water foot bath. Although warm water may initially feel better, cold water that has a few ice cubes added to it will help reduce inflammation and swelling of the feet. For best results, keep the feet immersed up to the ankles for 10 minutes, towel off, and then elevate the feet.

Prevention

- If you wear high heels, limit your time in them. Wear flat-heeled shoes to and from work.
- Measure both feet while standing on the metal sizing tray in the shoe store. If there is a difference in sizes, choose the larger size shoe and have a cotton heel liner added to the shoe on the smaller foot.
- The front of your shoes should be spacious enough for you to wiggle your toes and have up to a half-inch of clearance between your big toe and the front of the shoe. The heel should be snug, but not too tight.
- When buying shoes, shop late in the day when your feet are fully stretched out. Wear socks or stockings that you would normally wear with the shoes.

Cause for Concern

Aching feet may be symptomatic of other ailments that are best to rule out before beginning any home treatment. Cramping in the foot or leg, for example, can be caused by poor circulation brought on by atherosclerosis, the narrowing of the arteries that go to the legs. A doctor's exam and a medical prescription are needed for treatment.

Foot discomfort, diminished foot sensation, and infection can be symptoms of diabetes, which often develops during middle age. Contact your physician immediately if you suspect diabetes.

If the arch of the foot suddenly flattens out and the foot becomes swollen and painful, it's probably due to a degenerative stretching and subsequent collapse of the supporting tendons of the arch. Obesity is often a risk factor.

To be certain your foot has flattened, stand up straight with heels on the ground and feet facing forward. Have someone stand behind you and look at your feet. A flattened foot will project abnormally outward and make it look as if you have too many toes. It's necessary to see a doctor for an examination and treatment if your foot suddenly flattens.

If any foot problem doesn't seem to get better, or if it starts to feel worse despite home treatments, contact an orthopedist or podiatrist for an evaluation.

After a complete foot exam, an orthosis may be recommended. Made of fiberglass, flexible thermoplastic, foam, or leather, this custom-made device is either rigid or semi-rigid and is designed to keep your feet from moving abnormally when you walk or run. In theory, the orthosis limits movement or straightens the foot, thereby taking excessive pressure off the feet, ankle, knee, hip and back. Orthoses don't work for everyone, nor are they needed by everyone with sore feet. In some cases though, orthoses can clearly help to correct an arch-related problem.

WHAT TO DO

- Wear comfortable shoes.
- Limit your time in high heels if you choose to wear them.
- Switch to wider shoes if you have pain in the front of your foot or if you have a neuroma.
- Take pressure off the neuroma by cutting a hole through the insole of an athletic shoe.
- Wear over-the-counter arch supports when either an arch or both arches of the feet become sore or stiff.
- Give yourself a foot massage.
- Perform the "air alphabet" to stretch out your foot and ankle.
- Lie down and prop your feet up on some pillows to raise them higher than the level of your heart *but only if you don't have any vascular problems.*
- Lie down and keep the feet at heart level if you have a diagnosed vascular problem.
- Plunge your tired, aching feet into a cold water bath.
- Contact your physician immediately if you notice loss of sensation, numbness, or a tingling sensation in your feet.

Skin and Hair

GENERAL INFORMATION

The skin is the largest organ of the body. This complex, waterproof body sheath regulates internal temperature and, with its millions of nerve receptors, senses touch, external temperature, and pressure. Skin also provides a first line of defense against viruses, bacteria, fungi, and poisons. Skin may also provide signals about emotional and physical well-being.

The skin is composed of three layers: the epidermis, the dermis, and the subcutaneous tissue. The outermost epidermis has the thickness of a thin sheet of paper. Its cells are regulated all the time. As the cells die and fall off, they are replaced by cells that move up from lower skin levels.

The dermis, which holds the sweat glands and hair follicles, lies just below the epidermis. Sebaceous glands in this layer secrete sebum, or oil, through the hair follicles, and continually lubricate the skin. Perspiration, produced by the 2 million eccrine glands in the dermis, helps regulate intern body temperature.

Just below the dermis is the subcutaneous tissue, usually a layer of fat and connective tissue, which serves to insulate and protect the internal organs.

There are many skin and hair disorders, but only a few, such as malignant melanoma, a skin cancer, are life threatening. However, many cause both physical and motional difficulties. The skin's appearance may be altered by heredity, hygiene, medications, daily nutrition, insufficient rest and exercise, hormones, and sun exposure. If you are troubled by any skin disorder that appears to be spontaneous, or if home treatment fails to bring satisfactory results for a skin condition, consult a dermatologist.

SKIN CARE SPECIALISTS

DERMATOLOGIST (M.D.). A dermatologist is a medical doctor with additional training in the diagnosing and

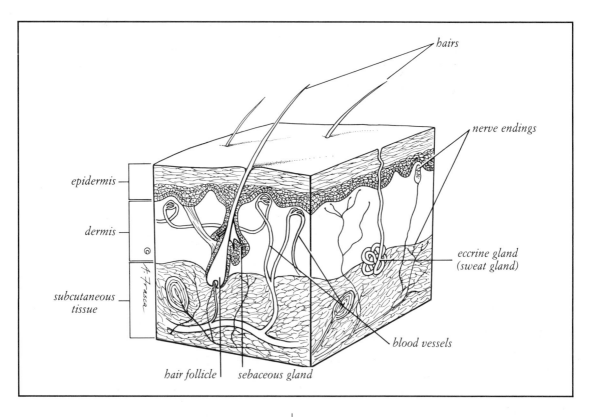

hairs

nerve endings

epidermis

dermis

eccrine gland
(sweat gland)

subcutaneous
tissue

blood vessels

hair follicle   sebaceous gland

treatment of disorders of the skin, hair, and nails. A dermatologist may perform surgery on benign and malignant growths, as well as correct cosmetic defects of the skin.

PHYSICIAN'S CARE REQUIRED

HUMAN BITE. When skin is torn and bleeding from a bite from human upper and lower teeth, the possibility of serious bacterial infection from saliva is great. Contact a physician or go to the hospital Emergency Department immediately for examination and treatment to prevent infection.

IMPETIGO. Quick-spreading, highly contagious bacterial skin infection com-

mon to babies and children, rarely adults. Symptoms include itchy, red patches that turn to pustules, crusting over to yellow sores. Responds well to antibiotics and clears within seven days.

SKIN CANCER. Basal cell and squamous cell carcinoma, and malignant melanoma are three forms of malignant cancer skin growths, mainly caused by exposure to ultraviolet radiation, genetics, X rays, or air pollution. Contact your physician immediately when you notice new or suspicious sores, lumps, or changes on the skin. May appear as red nodules, waxy bumps, or brown, flat flesh-colored lesion. Cure rate is high with early detection.

COMMON SKIN PROBLEMS

ACNE
Mild to severe skin eruption typified by red, inflamed bumps on the skin surface, excessively oily complexion, blackheads, and whiteheads. May cause permanent facial scarring. **Page 164**

BLISTERS
Common, fluid-filled bumps on the skin surface, caused by heat, cold, friction, or allergic reactions. **Page 166**

BOILS
A common bacterial infection of a hair follicle that develops into a pea-sized, pus-filled lump with a red, 9hiny surface. **Page 168**

BRUISES
Blood pools just below the surface of the skin following injury or disease, causing discoloration. Pain and swelling often accompany a moderate to severe impact injury. **Page 170**

BURNS
Skin damage from fire, heat, or chemicals, which may result in pain, swelling, blistering, nerve damage, and destruction. **Page 171**

CHAPPED SKIN
Dry, cracked, reddened, or roughened skin caused by lack of water in the skin. **Page 175**

COLD SORES
This common, highly contagious lesion is caused by the herpes virus and can arise on the lip or under the nose. When the blister ruptures, a painful white, red-ringed ulcer forms that finally scabs over and disappears within two weeks. **Page 177**

CUTS AND SCRAPES
Minimal blood loss and moderate skin damage are symptomatic of these oftentimes painful skin injuries. **Page 179**

continued

DANDRUFF
Mild flaking of the outer skin layers of the scalp, accompanied by occasional itching and redness. The smaller skin flakes may be matted together by oil. The problem is common, more cosmetic than medical, and easily treated.

Page 182

DRY SKIN
Scaly, brittle, and roughened skin, often accompanied by severe itching. The condition is aggravated during cold winter months, as well as by aging, but can occur in people in their forties as well. **Page 184**

ECZEMA
The collective group of specific noncontagious skin irritations that are typified by variable and intermittent itching, redness, oozing, and blistering are generally referred to as eczema. **Page 186**

HIVES
Swollen red skin patches triggered by an allergy to a substance, virus, insect bite, or stress. **Page 190**

INSECT BITES AND STINGS
Painful, usually temporary allergic skin reactions, accompanied by swelling, itching, and pain that can last for hours. In the case of anaphylactic shock and severe poisoning, immediate medical attention is required. Anaphylactic shock is an immediate and overwhelming allergic reaction leading to breathing and blood pressure problems, which can lead to death. **Page 193**

JOCK ITCH
A common contagious fungal, bacterial, and yeast infection of the groin. It is typified by itchy, red scaly skin patches on the groin, thighs, and buttocks. Often noted as a raised, red, scaling ring with a lightly colored center.

Page 195

LICE
Tiny, wingless parasites that feed on human blood, commonly in the pubic area and on the head. **Page 197**

POISON IVY
Nagging, unremitting intense itch and red rash from poison ivy resin. This later forms small yellow blisters and can take up to three weeks to clear.

Page 200

PSORIASIS
A chronic skin disorder manifested by plaques of dry, red, inflamed skin covered with silvery scales, generally found on elbows, knees, and scalp, as well as toenails and fingernails. It affects 1–5 percent of the American population and often requires medical attention.

Page 201

RAZOR BURN
A temporary skin irritation caused by shaving. Symptoms include florid red facial skin and tiny cuts. Eczema, ingrown hairs, and dry skin all can cause razor burn, but improper preparation of the beard for shaving is the main factor.

Page 204

SUNBURN
Reddened skin, localized pain, and blisters from too many unprotected hours in the sun. The long-term danger is potentially lethal skin cancer, which arises years after intense sun exposure.

Page 206

WARTS
This virus-caused skin disorder is mainly found on the fingers, hands, and soles of the feet and usually requires medical attention for removal.

Page 209

WRINKLES
Naturally occurring sagging skin layers due to aging, sun, and the effects of gravity.

Page 211

ACNE

Darrell E. Rigel, M.D.

Dr. Rigel is clinical associate professor of Dermatology at New York University Medical Center in New York City

Acne typically develops in adolescence and may continue into the early twenties. In fact, women can suffer until the mid-thirties before the triggering hormones finally settle down.

Eating too much sugar, not sleeping enough, too much sexual activity, and poor personal hygiene—often cited as causes for acne—are usually not. Even if you washed your face 100 times a day, it wouldn't prevent acne's skin eruptions. If you have a genetic tendency to acne, you will develop it no matter what you do.

Acne is an inflammation of the oil glands of the face that usually strikes during teenage years. This often psychologically distressing ailment begins with a small red bump on the surface of the skin. The inflammatory swelling around it usually causes the opening of the oil gland to be blocked, which causes sebum, the natural body oil that acts to retain moisture, to back up behind it. The surface of this plugged oil gland turns black when exposed to the air and develops what is called an open comedo, or a blackhead.

As the blackhead seals, bacteria breaks down the oil. The bacteria multiply and invade the surrounding tissue, and pus develops, creating a closed comedo, or whitehead. In laymen's terms this is a pimple. Researchers can't pinpoint acne's cause with any certainty. A genetic component is involved, however, and there is a hormonal component as well. Most dermatologists believe acne is triggered during adolescence when hormones change and the production of androgen, the male sex hormone, temporarily increases, stimulating both oil gland size and production. In women, the hormonal fluctuations that accompany monthly menstruation may set off an increase in acne.

There is also a stress component to acne, and again no one is sure why. People who are tense and under pressure tend to break out, perhaps because excess male hormones are released as part of the "fight or flight" response.

Shaving can cause a form of acne in African–American men especially, called pseudofollicutitis barbae (see RAZOR BURN, page 204). The hair follicles become irritated from the razor, and bumps develop on the hair follicles. The more frequently you shave, the more the follicles become irritated and raised, creating a vicious cycle. To prevent pseudofollicutitis barbae, stop shaving temporarily, even permanently in severe chronic cases, and apply a 0.5 percent hydrocortisone cream to help reduce the inflammation.

The use of birth control pills tends to improve acne, but problems may develop when a woman stops using the pills, because the resulting hormonal swings can cause acne. This is self-limiting and should clear up within six to eight months as the body accustoms itself to the new hormone level.

Treatment

Although acne can't be cured, mild acne can be successfully treated at home using daily preventive measures. Acne will not disappear overnight, but after two to three weeks of treatment, hopefully it will be 50 percent better.

Wash your face twice daily with warm soapy water. This cleansing clears debris from your skin and washes away bacteria that can lead to infectious acne. Don't waste money on facial "scrubs" available in the pharmacy. A washcloth and soap work just as well. Avoid strong soaps because they dry the skin and cause irritation. Mild soaps are sufficient in most cases. Experiment to find out which soap works best for your skin. Remember, the more sensitive your skin, the milder the soap for you.

If you develop blackheads or whiteheads, there are many OTC remedies that can help. Buy a product with benzoyl peroxide, a liquid commonly sold in either 5 percent or 10 percent solution. Start out with the weaker concentration. Before going to sleep at night, apply the medication to a clean washcloth and gently rub it over the affected areas. The benzoyl peroxide dries the skin, dissolves blackhead plugs, and kills some of the bacteria that lead to the inflammatory stage of acne.

You may find your skin is too sensitive when you use a 10 percent solution. Symptoms include reddened and dry skin. If that happens, use the medication every other day. Even a 5 percent solution may have this adverse reaction, so, again, switch to the alternate-day-treatment schedule.

When you have acne, you want to keep your face a little on the dry side. To ensure this, wipe your face once or twice a day with a washcloth lightly dipped in rubbing alcohol. The rubbing alcohol will tend to kill bacteria better than benzoyl peroxide, while the benzoyl peroxide is better for drying the acne and making it go away.

After several weeks, if neither the alcohol wipes nor the benzoyl peroxide works, try a 0.5 percent concentration of hydrocortisone cream that is available OTC. Apply the cream to the affected areas and gently rub it into the skin. This cream is especially effective against red, inflammatory acne.

Although the urge may be great, *do not squeeze* any whiteheads or blackheads. No matter how gently you try to squeeze or push, a certain percentage of your fingertip pressure goes to push the clogged material deeper into the pore. Instead of squeezing, dab benzoyl peroxide and dry out the area. In the long run, this helps prevent scarring that develops when bacteria is driven into the dermis and becomes inflamed.

Prevention

- Don't apply too much skin moisturizer or sunscreen. A thick layer of sunscreen can become a problem. Once you perspire under this lotion, sebum is prevented from leaving the pores, and acne can be aggravated.
- Makeup blocks the pores and starts the whole acne process. You may want to switch to oil-free cosmetics. (Water-based makeups still contain oil, so the key word to look for on labels is not "water-based," but "oil free.") You can use the oil-free makeup on a regular basis, but take it off at night before going to sleep.
- Wash your face with warm water and soap and be sure to rinse off all the soap residue when you're finished.

- Hair that covers the forehead and neck can block pores and bring on acne. Keep the hair short and avoid mousse or greasy hair preparations because they tend to clog the pores.

What the Doctor Will Do

When self-help measures fail, when acne is making you self-conscious, or when you're concerned that your acne may lead to permanent scarring, contact a dermatologist.

After closely examining your skin, the doctor may prescribe oral antibiotics such as tetracycline to be taken daily for two months or longer. Low dosage birth control pills (estrogen) may be prescribed for women with severe acne in order to suppress hormonal activity.

There is no such thing as a miracle cure for acne, but when medication is taken under a doctor's care, your complexion should clear sufficiently to prevent extreme self-consciousness or permanent scarring.

Over time, acne will vanish as mysteriously as it first appeared. Until then, wise management of the condition plus a good dose of patience is the best treatment available.

WHAT TO DO

- Wash your face twice daily with warm water and mild soap.
- Wash your face nightly with a 5 percent benzoyl peroxide acne preparation available OTC. For moderate to severe acne, use a 10 percent solution. If skin reddens or becomes too dry, use it on alternate nights.
- For red, inflammatory acne, apply a 0.5 percent hydrocortisone cream.
- Don't squeeze blackheads or whiteheads.
- When they must be used, apply *thin* layers of skin moisturizer and sunscreen to avoid clogging the pores.
- Keep hair away from the forehead and back of the neck. Do not use mousse or greasy hair preparations that may clog the pores of the forehead and neck.
- Contact a dermatologist if these measures don't work, if you feel extremely self-conscious about your appearance, or if you are afraid scarring may result.

BLISTERS

Earl E. Smith III, M.D.

Dr. Smith is chief of Emergency Services, Erlanger Medical Center, Chattanooga, Tennessee

If you injure the epidermis—the outer layer of skin—by rubbing it continuously, or suffer from allergic reactions to plants or insects, red, fluid-filled bumps called blisters can develop at the site. The liquid under the dead layer of skin is similar to blood plasma, minus the red cells, and will stay there until new skin forms underneath. Blisters are common, come in a variety of sizes, are often tender to the touch, and can develop anywhere on the body.

Treatment

Blisters should be treated differently, depending on their location. If one develops on the chest or forearm, areas that don't normally get bumped in the course of a day's activities, keep the blister covered with a clean dressing such as an adhesive bandage or gauze. Depending on the size of the blister, the body should reabsorb its liquid in three to seven days as new skin forms underneath.

If a blister develops in an area such as the hand, heel, elbow, or knee that can get rubbed during the day, then it's best to remove the fluid from the blister. To do this, take a sewing needle, hold it over a flame for 15 seconds to sterilize it, and then slowly insert it on the side of the blistered skin. Press down gently with your fingers to ease the fluid out of the opening. However, once the blister is open, the skin is left exposed and provides the perfect environment for bacteria to enter and cause an infection. For this reason, the dead skin "roof" of the blister must be removed. This allows two things to happen—the chance of infection is minimized and the exposed skin underneath will toughen up more quickly as it dries out in the air.

To remove the roof of a blister, take a washcloth, apply a mild soap, and while in either a bathtub or shower, gently rub the skin off. If this is too painful, then put the blistered area under cold, running water to numb the skin. You can also apply an ice cube for 5 minutes and then scrub off the skin gently with a washcloth and mild soap. Dry the area gently with a clean towel.

To prevent infection, clean the exposed area at least twice daily with warm water and mild soap.

The more a blister is left uncovered in a clean environment, the more quickly it will dry out, and new skin will develop. However, if the blister should become contaminated, apply an OTC antibiotic ointment to the blistered area and cover it with a bandage to prevent any dirt from being absorbed into the ointment. Remember that anytime you put an ointment on a blister, you slow down the drying and skin-thickening process, so only use antibiotics when absolutely necessary.

Prevention

- If you developed blisters on the hands after using tools or sports equipment, wear gloves.
- If blisters develop on your heels or toes, check your footwear for proper sizing or for any rough seams.
- Wear properly sized socks that won't move when you walk or run. If tube socks are the culprit, don't wear the one-size-fits-all models.
- Going sockless even in properly fitting shoes can cause blistering, so avoid this if you are prone to blisters.
- If you are involved in a sports activity, make sure your shoes are dry and not still damp or wet from previous use.

Cause for Concern

If you start to notice increasing redness around any blister, with tenderness or warmth to the touch, or if pus develops that is accompanied by red streaks, this means infection has set in. If this happens —and it usually does only when you have a very large blister—take acetaminophen, aspirin, or ibuprofen tablets according to instructions on the bottle to reduce fever, pain, and inflammation symptoms. Also, increase the frequency of washing with soap and water to three to four times daily. Dry the area with a clean towel and then apply a light layer of an OTC antibacterial ointment.

If there is no improvement after two days, contact your physician. The doctor may prescribe a stronger antibacterial ointment in addition to systemic antibiotic medication.

WHAT TO DO

- Keep blister protected with a bandage if it's in an area that may get bumped or jostled during the day.
- With a sterilized needle, rupture a large blister, or rupture any blister that has the potential to be rubbed often during the day.
- After expressing the fluid from a blister, remove its roof by rubbing it gently with a washcloth, warm water, and mild soap. If too painful, numb the area first with cold running water or an ice cube.
- Apply a light layer of antibiotic ointment and cover with a bandage if there is any danger of contamination.
- Clean the area twice daily with warm water and mild soap to prevent infection.
- Take preventive measures to avoid blisters. Wear gloves when necessary, make sure shoes and socks fit properly, and don't wear damp or wet shoes for sports activity.

Signs of infection include increasing redness around the blister, the area becomes warm or hot to the touch, or pus or red streaks develop in the blister. To treat the infection, do the following:

- Wash the area three to four times daily with mild soap and warm water.
- Apply an antibacterial ointment.
- Take acetaminophen, aspirin, or ibuprofen to reduce resulting pain, inflammation, or fever symptoms.
- If there is no improvement after two days, contact your physician.

BOILS

Jerome Z. Litt, M.D.

Dr. Litt is assistant clinical professor of Dermatology, Case Western Reserve University School of Medicine in Cleveland, Ohio

A boil, or furuncle, is a common skin condition that is caused when bacteria on the skin, usually staphylococci, grow in the oil gland of a hair follicle. Once germs proliferate in the oil gland, a localized infection and inflammation of the skin begin rapidly. Fever may sometimes develop. As the skin tissue swells, a small, red, tender lump, the size of a pea, emerges.

If left untreated, a boil can reach *enormous* size in a matter of days. Pus, formed by the white blood cells that fight the infection, fills the boil and puts it under extreme pressure. The top surface then becomes shiny and extremely painful. Once the boil bursts, pain diminishes, and healing begins.

Treatment

A boil on any body part except the face, can often be treated effectively at home using hot, wet compresses.

To make a compress, take a cotton cloth—a folded cotton handkerchief, or pieces of bed linen folded eight layers thick. Dip this into hot Pedi-Boro solution, an antiseptic, and gently wring it out. (To make Pedi-Boro solution, dissolve the contents of one Pedi-Boro Soak Pak in a pint of hot water. These packets are available OTC in the pharmacy.) Gently pat the infected area—on and off, for 10 minutes—remoistening the cloth when necessary. Repeat the process three times a day.

This compress will help relieve pain and swelling, bring the infection to a head, and cause the boil to rupture and the pus to drain.

Do not squeeze a boil with your fingers. This may force the infected matter deeper into the skin. The boil should be kept scrupulously clean with antibacterial soap. If there are any germs on the skin surface, the boil can recur at the same spot and furunculosis—a chronic condition—can develop.

Cause for Concern

For a boil on the face above the lips, on the nose, or in the ear, seek medical attention immediately. Boils in these areas are extremely dangerous because of their tendency to seep and drain directly into the brain, which can result in infection. The doctor will lance the boil to drain the pus and prescribe antibiotics to kill the bacteria.

If a fever accompanies your boil, or if you have recurring boils, consult your physician. If the boil contains fluid, the doctor will lance it to allow the pus to come out. Antibiotics—usually erythromycin—are prescribed. If the boil is large, the medication should be taken for several weeks. For smaller boils, ten to fourteen days are generally sufficient.

A carbuncle is not to be confused with a furuncle, or boil. A carbuncle is a tremendous boil, or a series of boils, that join together and grow sideways. Carbuncles, which usually develop on the back of the neck, are severe infections, larger, deeper, and more extensive and painful than boils, and their germs can spread via the bloodstream. Consult your physician for treatment.

WHAT TO DO

- Dip a folded cotton handkerchief or pieces of bed linen folded in eight layers into hot Pedi-Boro solution.
- Pat the infected area on and off for 10 minutes. Repeat the process three times daily until the boil ruptures, and pus drains.
- Keep the area clean with antibacterial soap and water.
- If you have a high fever that accompanies a boil, or if the boil is on your face, or if you have recurring boils, see your physician for treatment.

- A carbuncle is a boil, only larger, deeper, more painful and extensive, and usually found on the back of the neck.

Consult your physician for proper treatment.

BRUISES

Bruce E. Katz, M.D.

Dr. Katz is an assistant clinical professor at the College of Physicians and Surgeons, Columbia University, and director, Dermatologic Cosmetic Surgery Clinic, Columbia–Presbyterian Medical Center in New York City

A bruise results from a pooling of blood which can occur when blood vessels have been damaged by trauma or disease; after receiving a blood transfusion; or after taking certain medications such as aspirin, asthma bronchodilators, and antidepressants. The discoloration that appears on the skin is actually blood that has settled in the area just below the skin surface and above the muscle.

Bruises appear first as reddish tinges shortly after an impact injury, but change to black/blue hues before finally turning greenish-yellow as the blood slowly reabsorbs back into the body.

Treatment

The best way to ease pain and swelling, and lessen potential discoloration to the skin after an injury is to apply an ice pack to the injury site as soon as possible. The cold stops internal bleeding from the damaged blood vessels and causes the blood vessels to constrict. The more blood that collects after an injury, the more pronounced the bruise will be, and the longer it will take to disappear.

To make an ice pack, fill a plastic bag with ice and pour in at least a cupful of cold water to speed up the cold dispersal. Seal the bag and place it over a clean moist towel directly on the injury site. Hold it there for intervals of 15 minutes on, 15 minutes off, over the next twenty-four hours. If you don't have any ice available, use a cold can of soda or frozen juice container.

After twenty-four hours, apply heat to the area in order to promote healing by increasing local circulation. Heat can be in the form of a hot bath, shower, hot tub, heating pad, or whirlpool. Warm the damaged area for 15-minute intervals several times a day.

Any swelling that accompanies a bruise can be minimized by elevating the damaged area above the level of the heart for at least 15 minutes following injury. This causes blood to flow away from the injury site, helping to minimize the swelling.

For any minor discomfort and pain resulting from the injury, take acetaminophen or ibuprofin tablets according to label directions. Avoid aspirin because it thins the blood, causing more swelling.

Cause for Concern

When bruises appear on the body for no apparent reason, have them checked immediately by a physician because they could be symptomatic of different diseases, including aplastic anemia, hemophilia, and leukemia.

These illness-related bruises generally show up in areas that tend to be traumatized more easily, such as the hands, knees, and forearms. Bruising can also appear in the soft palate of the mouth. When bruises appear under the fingernails and toenails, this may be a warning sign of an early melanoma, and should be evaluated by a physician. If detected and treated early enough, the potentially lethal melanoma can be successfully treated.

Anytime you are struck in the eye (see BLACK EYE, page 14), you are at risk for serious eye injury. The colorful bruising of the skin around the eye, often called a "shiner," is typical after impact in this region, but it's the potentially damaging effect of the impact on the eye itself that has to be evaluated. Contact your ophthalmologist for a complete examination immediately.

WHAT TO DO

- Apply an ice pack as soon as possible to the area to stop internal bleeding and cause blood vessels to constrict. Use the ice in 15-minute on-off intervals.
- To speed up the recovery process, after twenty-four hours apply heat in the same 15-minute intervals. A hot bath, shower, heating pad, or whirlpool all work well.
- To minimize swelling that often accompanies a bruise, keep the damaged body part elevated above the heart.
- For pain relief, take 2 acetaminophen or ibuprofen tablets.
- If bruises appear spontaneously on the body without trauma, they could be symptomatic of underlying disease. Contact your physician for an evaluation.

BURNS

John C. Johnson, M.D.

Dr. Johnson is the director of the Center for Emergency and Trauma Care at Porter Memorial Hospital, Valparaiso, Indiana, and the former president of the American College of Emergency Physicians

When something hotter than your skin touches it, you get burned. Symptoms include redness of the skin, pain, swelling, blistering, and in the case of severe burns, charred skin, nerve damage, and destruction.

Burns are classified by degree:
- A first-degree burn is superficial and affects the outermost portion of the skin, and its symptoms can include reddening of the skin, pain, and sometimes swelling. Pain will diminish within two days. Typical first-degree burns come from sunburn or quickly touching a hot cooking implement.
- A second-degree burn can affect either

the outer layer of skin in mild cases, or portions of the second skin layer, the dermis, in more severe cases. Symptoms include skin redness, pain, swelling, and some blisters. A burn from scalding grease or water is a typical example. Second-degree burns are probably the most painful because the burn damages but doesn't kill surrounding nerves.

If small, most second-degree burns can be treated at home. After treatment, pain will diminish in two to three days, but won't be gone completely until new skin surface has built back up. For a small burn, this could be three days, and a week to ten days for a burn over a larger area.

- Third-degree burns destroy all skin layers and penetrate deep below the skin surface. The damaged skin may be white, red, brown, tan, or charred (black) in color. There is no blistering. Swelling may be extensive, and since there is extensive nerve damage, there is no pain and generally no bleeding.

Treatment

The seriousness of a burn is a function of the temperature of heat involved and how long the skin was in contact with it. The longer that intense heat is applied to the skin, the more serious a burn will be.

The trick in treating a burn is to reduce the high temperature by immediately reversing the flow of heat back to the point of initial skin contact. Heat will continue to flow through your tissues causing a deeper burn only until the flow is reversed. To stop the flow, apply a cold liquid to the burn as quickly as possible.

I had a young boy as a patient who had been severely scalded by chicken grease he had spilled out of a frying pan. His quick-thinking mother immediately doused the burn with a gallon of milk that was sitting on the counter and the boy came away with almost no burn at the point of contact, just a faint redness that was similar to a sunburn.

For best results, plunge the burned area into cold water, or hold it under running cold water until the pain diminishes and the skin is no longer hot. However, do not use ice water or ice unless that is all that's available. In some cases, this severe cold may result in further skin or nerve damage beyond that of the burn.

For chemical burns, immediately rinse the skin with a steady flow of water from a shower or hose to remove contaminants. Fifteen minutes or more of rinsing may be required to neutralize some chemicals.

If you are wearing polyester fiber clothing and it catches fire, the material can melt into a ball and stick to your skin. Although you may immediately put out the flame, you must continue to cool off the polyester or tar goo with cold water. Whether you try to get the goo off yourself depends on how easy it is to remove. If you begin to peel layers of skin off with the material, then leave it alone. Emergency Department physicians have a number of effective solvents available.

After the pain of a first-degree burn has diminished with cold water, gently dry the area. Apply a light dressing of antibiotic cream. Not only will this be soothing, but it will keep the wound moist and protect it from infection. Do not apply butter to any burn, no matter how minor. Butter doesn't do anything for a burn, except cause infection.

Never apply ointments to a burn. Ointments are similar to grease and will trap heat and not allow moisture to move back and forth from the wound. In some cases, ointment can actually make a burn worse by harboring the body's own heat, thereby forcing it deeper into the tissues and causing more damage.

You don't need prescription medications to get substantial pain relief. Take 2 aspirin or ibuprofen tablets (200 mgs) every four hours if you are not allergic and don't have a sensitive stomach. Both medications inhibit the release of chemicals that result in pain. If you can't tolerate either aspirin or ibuprofen, take 2 acetaminophen tablets, but the pain-relief effects will be less pronounced.

Blisters are common in moderate to severe second-degree burns. A blister is the watery protein fluid from the body. Blisters form a padding over the burned area, which provides protection from further injury. Blisters often don't appear right away, but may develop six to eighteen hours later. A delayed-onset blister indicates a deeper second-degree burn, and medical assistance is recommended.

If you have a small blister, leave it alone and in a day or so it will go down in size and be reabsorbed by the body. For larger blisters, the size of a dime or bigger, or for blisters in areas that are likely to be broken by activity—knees, fingers, elbows, or feet —it's best to drain them.

To drain a small blister, take a clean sewing needle and heat it in a flame to sterilize it. Clean the skin and the needle with rubbing alcohol and let the alcohol dry. Stick the corner of the blister with the needle and express the fluid out. Unfortunately, bacteria usually develops in blisters that have been deflated, so the loose skin must be removed in order to expose the injured skin to the antibiotic cream.

Once the roof of the blister has been removed, apply an antibacterial cream to keep the skin moist, allow fluid to move in and out of tissue, and protect the wound from infection. Once you apply the cream, cover it with a sterile gauze bandage.

Change the dressing twice a day. Once the new skin begins to form, stop applying the cream, and as long as it won't be traumatized or get dirty by daily activity, you may leave the bandage off and expose the damaged area to air. To keep the skin soft and comfortable as it continues to heal, apply a small amount of skin moisturizer as needed.

Cause for Concern

Although most first- and minor second-degree burns can be treated successfully at home, third-degree burns require immediate medical attention. Also, large burns and burns that develop fairly large blisters also require medical care.

Flash burns to the face from an explosion need to be checked in the Emergency Department. Often facial swelling and burns to the mouth, nose, or airway are involved. The airway can swell shut and the patient asphyxiate. A first-degree burn will cause the lips and eyes to swell, while a second-degree burn may close the lips, mouth, and eyes.

If you've been involved in a fire in an enclosed area—one that takes place in a shed or workroom, for example—seek medical attention. The airways could be burned and swollen. Typical symptoms include a persistent hacking cough and difficulty in breathing. A tube may have to be inserted in the airway to assist breathing.

When hot or burning particles become stuck to the skin, this creates a bacterial pathway into the body, and I can almost guarantee that you will develop a bacterial infection. Contact your physician. He will most likely prescribe oral antibiotics.

If the skin doesn't break down that much after a burn, you're not going to have much worry about infection. However, once the flow of temperature has been reversed with a cold liquid, any skin surface damaged by a burn is no longer impenetrable to bacteria or chemicals. Measures must be taken to protect the skin from infection.

Damaged skin doesn't have good circulation and has difficulty fighting off infection. For people who have serious complications from burns, problems won't always be apparent on the first day, but may surface several days or even weeks later when infection has taken hold. Therefore, anything you can do to lessen the amount of tissue damage will decrease the potential problems of infection.

When burn sites become infected, seek medical attention. Signs of infection include a beefy red color and pain that becomes progressively worse over days. You may also notice pus in the blisters, and the burn site will have a foul, usually cheesy or fruity odor. A low-grade temperature of 99–100.5 degrees is also common.

What the Doctor Will Do

After examination, a physician will clean and dress the wound, and may prescribe oral antibiotics.

WHAT TO DO

- Apply a cold liquid to the burn as quickly as possible to reverse the flow of heat back to the original point of contact. *Don't* use ice water or ice.
- Don't apply butter to a burn; it may lead to infection.
- If polyester or other material melts onto your skin, cool it off with cold running water before attempting to remove it. If you can't get it off easily, head to the hospital Emergency Department.
- After using cold water to diminish burn pain, apply a light OTC antibiotic cream.
- Don't use ointments on burns. They don't allow moisture to penetrate and can increase the severity of a burn.
- Take 2 aspirin or ibuprofen tablets (200 mgs) every four hours if you are not allergic or your stomach is not overly sensitive. Use acetaminophen if you are under twelve or can't tolerate aspirin or ibuprofen.
- For a moderate size blister, prick the edge with a sterilized needle, and express the liquid.
- Remove the entire roof of the blister (deflated skin) and apply a bacterial cream to keep this exposed area moist and speed healing. Cover with a sterile gauze bandage.
- If burned skin or surrounding tissue becomes infected, seek medical attention.

CHAPPED SKIN

Stephen B. Kurtin, M.D.

Dr. Kurtin is professor of Dermatology, Mount Sinai Hospital, New York City

Low humidity and low temperature are the major causes of chapped skin. These two climatic factors, when coupled with wind, will literally suck water right out of the skin, wrinkling and drying, and causing it to turn leathery.

Treatment

The best way to prevent chapped skin is to keep water from escaping the skin, and this means using a moisturizer on a regular basis. A moisturizing cream or lotion does *not* add moisture to the skin. However, when applied to damp or wet skin, it helps retain the existing water.

Despite advertising hype, there is not one magic cream or lotion that will revitalize skin, and high price does not necessarily ensure a better product. If the moisturizer you use costs half the price of another one, but still does the job for you, continue to use it.

To apply a moisturizer, after a shower or bath pat yourself lightly with a towel so your skin is moist but not wet, and then rub a light layer of moisturizer over it.

Experiment with moisturizers to find the one you like. If the moisturizer feels greasy and oily, then it's too heavy for your skin. Conversely, if your skin still feels dry after applying moisturizing cream, then it's too light.

Petroleum jelly is certainly not an elegant product, but it's fine for moisturizing your skin. Apply a light layer to chapped skin and gently rub it in. To avoid staining clothes, gently wipe off any excess with a tissue.

Washing dishes can also lead to chapped hands. The cause isn't hot water, but the soaps and dishwashing detergents. The soaps and detergents remove oils from the skin.

When washing dishes, wear rubber gloves with a separate pair of thin cotton gloves underneath them. The cotton gloves help retain moisture in the hands. Also, when the cotton gloves become dirty, they are easy to wash and use again. You can't do this if you buy cotton-lined rubber gloves.

Don't use extremely hot water when you wash dishes. This speeds up the removal of essential skin oils and the high temperature can also irritate the skin.

When you are finished washing the dishes, pat your hands lightly with a cloth and then apply a moisturizer while the skin is still damp.

If you are prone to dry, chapped hands from simply washing your hands, switch to a mild hand soap. The best mild soaps on the market contain moisturizing cream, or are special brands that are labeled "super fatted." There are more expensive moisturizing hand soaps available, but the brand that tests as good as any, and is cheaper, is Dove.

Although some doctors recommend home humidifiers, especially in the winter when houses are drier and overheated, I don't find them to be all that helpful in the prevention or treatment of chapped, dry skin. In my view, humidifiers are not large enough to put out the amount of moisture into the air that your skin actually needs.

Skin may also be irritated by friction and abrasion, such as rubbing the skin against rough clothing, or, as is the case with exercisers, rubbing the skin of one inner thigh against the other. This may cause a painful irritation that stings or burns the skin.

Natural smooth-fiber clothing as a rule is softer on the skin than synthetic counterparts, so if your skin chapping problem stems from your clothing, switch to a cotton or silk wardrobe. Also, after washing, make sure your clothing is completely rinsed of all detergent residue. In some cases, it may help to run the clothing through the rinse cycle a second time.

To prevent skin under your arms, in your groin, and between your thighs from being chapped while exercising, apply a thin layer of petroleum jelly before you start any vigorous activity. The skin areas will rub smoothly over each other without chapping. Take the ointment with you and reapply as needed.

Cause for Concern

If your skin becomes dry, cracked, red, and painful after washing dishes, this is a sign of irritant contact eczema, a skin ailment (see ECZEMA, page 186) caused by a chemical irritant in the detergent. Call a dermatologist for an examination and treatment. A topical corticosteroid ointment or cream may be prescribed to reduce inflammation and moisturize the damaged skin.

If your dry hands do not respond to basic moisturizing methods, apply an OTC hydrocortisone cream several times daily. However, most difficult dry skin cases require stronger hydrocorticone formulations that can only be prescribed by a physician.

Chapped Lips

Like chapped skin, chapped lips are caused by lack of moisture in the skin. The lips typically become dry from low humidity. But by rubbing your tongue over them, you cause them to dry out even more, which in turn causes the lips to crack, peel, and to become unsightly, and painful.

Snow and sand are both great reflectors of sun, which can burn the lips and lead to chapping. Dry mountain air will also speed the loss of moisture in the lips by drying them and eventually lead to chapping. If you know that you will be going to the mountains to ski or spending time at the beach, plan ahead to anticipate any problems.

Treatment

Many products on the market are formulated specifically for chapped lips. However, a good lip product should completely coat the lips and stay on for extended periods.

I happen to like Carmex and Lipmedex, two OTC products that do a very good job of keeping the lips moist. A light coating of petroleum jelly also works fine. Lipstick also helps prevent chapped lips and moisturizes lips that have become chapped.

Cause for Concern

In some extreme cases, the lips may also become infected. If you develop pustules on the lips, or have an open or cracked sore that oozes liquid, contact your dermatologist for an examination and treatment.

Prevention

- Moisturize your skin and lips before going out.
- Use special sun-protective lipsticks available in the pharmacy. These clear lipsticks moisturize the lips and prevent chapping. Since they also contain sun block, they keep the lips from getting sunburned as well. Reapply the lipstick throughout the day in order to maximize your protection.

WHAT TO DO

- Use a moisturizing lotion or cream regularly.

- Wear special rubber gloves and a separate pair of thin cotton glove liners when washing the dishes.
- Don't use extremely hot water when washing dishes.
- Pat hands lightly with a cloth so hands remain moist and apply moisturizer after washing your hands or the dishes.
- Use a mild hand soap.
- Apply a thin layer of moisturizer before vigorous activity to protect the skin under your arms, groin, and thigh from irritation.
- Use OTC lip moisturizers that completely coat the lips and stay on for extended periods.
- Wear sun-blocking lipsticks if you plan to snow-ski or spend time at the beach.
- If your skin becomes cracked, reddened, and painful, or if you develop pustules or sores on your lips, contact a dermatologist for an examination and treatment.

COLD SORES

Hillard H. Pearlstein, M.D.

Dr. Pearlstein is assistant clinical professor of Dermatology, Mount Sinai School of Medicine, New York City

Cold sores, also called fever blisters, and known medically as herpes simplex virus 1, are a common and notoriously recurring nuisance. Symptoms include blisters on the lip, under the nose, sometimes fever. A cold sore usually clears by itself in seven to twelve days, and rarely leads to any medical complications. The cold sore virus is highly contagious and easily transmitted in saliva or close sexual or social contact.

Some people may get a cold sore once in their life, others may get them once a year, while others may have them once every three weeks.

The initial herpes infection typically occurs before the age of four without any cold-sore symptoms exhibited. The virus lies dormant in the nervous system, sometimes for years, until it is triggered by one of three major factors. Extreme sun exposure from the beach, sunbathing, or skiing in particular seems to precipitate cold sores in many cases. Upper respiratory infection accompanied with or without a fever also results in the classic lip blister, hence the name "cold sore" or "fever blister." Emotional stress can also trigger cold sores.

Any reactivation of oral herpes is usually, but not always, signaled twenty-four to forty-eight hours prior to an outbreak by an itching or tingling sensation in the lips. A small red area develops, followed by a blister or group of tiny blisters that fills with liquid. When this blister ruptures, the area scabs over and eventually disappears.

Treatment

Although there is no effective cure for cold sores, there are several remedies that can relieve symptoms.

If sun exposure triggers your cold sores, avoid direct exposure on the face. If you go to the beach, sunbathe, or ski, apply a sun block to your lips. The sun block should have a UV-A rating no lower than 25.

Ice applied directly to the cold sore site prior to the eruption of a blister can reduce the potential swelling. Wrap an ice cube in a damp washcloth and keep it on the area for 5 minutes. Reapply it every hour. I don't recommend icing the area for longer periods because the skin is very thin on the lip and extreme cold may lead to frostbite damage.

Any drying or astringent OTC cold sore preparation that contains camphor and/or phenol such as Campho-Phenique

or Orabase may provide relief if applied in the early stages. When used in the scab stage, these ointments can help prevent painful cracking and bleeding.

A light coating of petroleum jelly to the scab to keep it from cracking and bleeding also works well to reduce pain. A topical OTC antibiotic ointment such as Neosporin or Bactine may help prevent secondary bacterial infection. Apply it according to directions.

To speed healing, don't touch or pick at cold sore scabs. For any pain and fever discomfort, take aspirin, acetaminophen, or ibuprofen.

What the Doctor Will Do

If you suffer persistent outbreaks of cold sores, contact your dermatologist. There is now a prescription antiviral medication called acyclovir that won't permanently cure you of cold sores, but may help limit or even abort them if taken early enough.

Acyclovir comes as an ointment, but I find it does not work as well as the oral capsules. Both medications are taken five times a day for five days. When the capsules are taken on a daily basis for chronic cases, acyclovir may aid in preventing recurrence.

WHAT TO DO

- Avoid direct and prolonged sun exposure to the face.
- Apply a total protection sunblock to the lips and nostril area when outside for long periods in the sun.
- Apply an ice cube wrapped in a wash-

cloth to the site for 5-minute intervals as soon as you first notice any tingling or numbness in your lip.

- Use an OTC cold sore preparation containing camphor and/or phenol regularly to aid in drying the cold sore.
- Apply a light coating of petroleum jelly to the scab to keep it from cracking and bleeding.
- Don't touch or pick at the scab.
- Take acetaminophen or ibuprofen for pain or fever relief.
- For persistent outbreaks of cold sores, contact your dermatologist.

CUTS AND SCRAPES

Barry Zide, D.M.D., M.D.

Dr. Zide is an associate professor of Plastic Surgery at the New York University Medical Center in New York City

Minor Cuts

When you've been cut, it's important to know how you got cut. If a foreign body such as sand, grit, or a small pebble gets into the cut, this may lead to infection or "tattooing"—the permanent discoloration of the skin caused by foreign matter left in the healing wound. Therefore, it's important that all wounds be properly cleaned and dressed.

The cleanliness of the wound—and the cutting object—are also critical to the healing time after injury. For example, if you got cut while paddling in a swamp, there's certainly a good possibility for infection. However, if you got cut with a kitchen knife you were removing from the dishwasher—probably as clean a cut as I could make with my scalpel—the chance for infection is much less.

Treatment

In 99 out of 100 cases, the most effective way to treat a minor cut is to apply direct pressure to the area to stop the flow of blood. Blood takes a while to clot, so this means holding or pressing down on the cut for 5 to 10 minutes.

Gauze or a clean cloth is excellent to hold on the wound and absorb the blood as you press. When either the gauze or cloth becomes soaked with blood, do not remove it, but place another clean dressing directly on top and reapply pressure.

For very superficial cuts, I like my teabag remedy the best. Take an ordinary moistened tea bag and press it down gently on the wound. Hold it there until the bleeding stops. Tea has tannic acid in it, and when this mixes with the blood from the wound, it helps the blood to coagulate quickly.

Do not apply a tourniquet of any type when you have a cut. You risk the chance of extensive nerve and tissue damage by stopping the flow of blood to the site. Direct pressure will work in all cases, except where a major artery has been severed and considerable amounts of blood gush or spurt out.

If the cut begins to bleed again, reapply pressure. Apply a dressing and go to your doctor or hospital's Emergency Department if you think you might need stitches.

To keep dirt out and protect the cut from reopening, apply a sterile rectangular adhesive bandage so there is slight pressure against the cut. With most minor cuts, healing should be complete in seven to ten days.

Don't apply any ointments or antiseptic sprays to a cut. The body's own immune system will effectively stave off any infection and these first-aid products are of little value.

What the Doctor Will Do

Most minor cuts can be treated at home. However, the direction of a cut is an important factor in how the skin will eventually heal.

If I make an elective incision on the face along the wrinkle lines, the scar tends not to show very much. But if I cut 90 degrees to the wrinkle lines, the scar will be more noticeable even if the closure method is identical. If either you or your child falls and receives a vertical cut to the forehead, contact a plastic surgeon or go to the local hospital's Emergency Department for treatment to reduce your chances of visible scarring.

If you do need stitches, it's best to have the stitching done during what I call the "golden period." For any cuts to the face, this period is about twelve hours, but may be extended by early cleaning. However, both hand and lower extremity cuts should be stitched within six hours in order to eliminate the risk of infection and ensure proper healing.

Minor Scrapes

The skin has several different layers, but when you fall on a hard or jagged surface, you generally scrape off the epidermis, the outer protective skin layer that is needed to repel water and germs. Scrapes are often a minor injury, but if the abrasion affects a large portion of skin, or if any grit or foreign matter becomes embedded in the scrape, there is a risk of infection, tattooing, and scarring.

Treatment

After an accident, you need to look carefully at your scrape. In the absence of severe bleeding, start to clean the wound. To remove any debris effectively, use cold running water and gently wipe the area with a clean washcloth. In many cases, this is sufficient cleansing. However, for deeply embedded grit and gravel, you should thoroughly scrub the area soon after your accident or else the skin will become permanently tattooed when it heals.

To remove deeply embedded foreign matter, take an ice cube or ice pack and numb the area for 3 to 5 minutes. When the abrasion is totally iced and sufficiently numb, use a clean, moist, and soapy washcloth and vigorously rub the area. Shampoo can be used in place of soap. Both the soap and shampoo act as solvents to remove the dirt.

Bright red blood will ooze from capillaries in the area. When all the dirt is out, reapply the ice to relieve pain symptoms, and pat the scrape dry with a sterile gauze pad or cloth. Apply some OTC antibacterial ointment and cover with a nonstick pad. Ibuprofen and acetaminophen can be taken for pain relief.

The secret in treating a scrape is in dressing the abrasion after it's been cleaned. Many people make the mistake of covering up the scrape with a bandage and allowing a scab to form. A scab is composed of dried blood and superficial dermis layers of skin and plays no role in promoting healing.

The key to recovery is always to keep the damaged area moist, but not with water. After the scrape has been adequately cleaned and dried, apply ordinary petroleum jelly, or else a light layer of an OTC antibiotic ointment such as Bacitracin or Polysporin. Use these ointments for the first two to three days but no longer, because allergies to the ointment occur frequently. Neosporin ointment causes allergic reactions in 15–20 percent of people, typical symptoms being pustules, skin redness, and itching. I don't recommend its use.

I do recommend Neutrogena hand cream for all minor abrasions. It does a good job of moisturizing the wound. I squeeze out a generous dose and rub it gently over the abrasion. A nonadherent gauze pad is then placed over the area to make sure the medication does not rub off, and this is held in place with tape.

Bandages should be changed two to three times daily and ointment or lotion reapplied. As an alternative to taking off the bandage each time, just lift up the edge of the bandage and squirt new ointment in.

Within twenty-four hours, take off the bandage and wash the area with mild soap and water, or baby shampoo. Whatever you do, don't take a bath in order to clean the wound, because the dirty, soapy bath water can quickly bring on infection.

Cause for Concern

For deep, long, or jagged cuts, or if you have difficulty moving some muscles—which is a sign of nerve damage—or if the pain level increases the next day instead of decreases, head to the hospital Emergency Department for treatment.

Infection can easily develop if you fail to use an antibiotic ointment and don't wash the area regularly. Signs of infection include redness extending out from the wound to unaffected areas, fever, swelling, warmth, increased oozing, or pus. Contact your doctor for further treatment if you have any of these symptoms.

If you're in extreme pain, or if your abrasion is quite deep, head to the hospital Emergency Department. You will be given a local anesthetic, and a doctor will use a surgical scrub brush or a toothbrush to clean the area completely. If you haven't had a tetanus shot in the preceding five years, you will be given a booster shot to immunize you against *Clostridium tetani,* a bacterium that is found in dirt. Introducing this organism into the body with a cut, scrape, or puncture wound can lead to tetanus, an infection that causes painful muscle contractions, lockjaw, and eventually death if left untreated.

WHAT TO DO

- Apply direct pressure to minor cuts to stop the flow of blood. This may take upward of 10 minutes.
- Use a gauze pad or clean cloth and press it over the cut to absorb the blood.
- To speed blood coagulation, apply an ordinary moistened tea bag to the cut and press lightly until the bleeding stops.

- Don't apply a tourniquet when you have a cut.
- When blood flow stops, clean the cut and surrounding area with a clean cloth and water, making sure to get out all embedded dirt.
- Don't apply any antiseptic sprays or ointments.
- Apply a sterile adhesive bandage to the cut.
- Consult your doctor or proceed to the hospital Emergency Department for treatment if your cut is deep, long, or jagged. If you perceive any numbness, or a muscle can't be moved normally, which is a sign of nerve damage, contact your physician.
- For longer or complicated cuts on the face, consult a plastic surgeon for early treatment. This may reduce chances of permanent scarring.
- When you scrape yourself and the skin bleeds, use cold running water and gently wipe the area clean with a cloth.
- For deeply embedded dirt and grit, numb the area for 3–5 minutes with an ice cube or ice pack. Apply mild soap or shampoo to a moist washcloth and vigorously rub the area to remove particles. Reapply ice when finished to numb the pain.
- If this process is too painful, or if you can't remove all the grit, head to the hospital Emergency Department.
- To prevent scabs and speed up new skin growth, apply a thin layer of petroleum jelly to the scrape. Apply a nonadhesive gauze pad over this and tape it in place. Reapply the jelly two to three times daily. Bacitracin or Polysporin may be used in place of petroleum jelly, but *only* for the first two or three days. With continued use, allergic reactions frequently develop to these ointments.
- Wash the area within twenty-four hours with a mild soap or baby shampoo and water. After each washing, reapply the petroleum jelly and gauze bandaging.

DANDRUFF

Robert L. Rietschel, M.D.

Dr. Rietschel is clinical associate professor of Dermatology at both LSU and Tulane University Medical Centers, and chairman of the Department of Dermatology at the Ochsner Clinic in New Orleans, Louisiana

Most people at some point in their lives will have simple dandruff, the flaking of the outer layers of dead skin on the scalp, which may be accompanied by mild itching. The problem is usually cosmetic, not medical, and can be treated successfully with very basic home measures.

Treatment

The most successful treatment for dandruff —for most people with dandruff—is daily shampooing. By shampooing frequently, you remove excessive scale buildup and decrease the microorganisms that grow in the scales and contribute to some of the inflammatory symptoms you may have.

Although some people have grown up with the idea that washing their hair every day is harmful, this isn't the case with the gentle, scientifically formulated shampoos of today.

For people who only shampoo once a week, dandruff will be extremely difficult to control. I recommend shampooing at *least* twice weekly.

If the daily use of regular shampoos containing either sodium lauryl sulfate, sodium laureth sulfate, or ammonium laureth sulfate does not relieve the symptoms, or if your dandruff is moderate to severe, then switch to a specially formulated medicated dandruff shampoo available in your pharmacy or supermarket. The key anti-dandruff ingredients to look for are zinc pyrithione, sulfur, salicylic acid, coal tar, and selenium sulfide.

Although your hair won't have the nice feel that you get from the more elegant detergent shampoos, these dandruff mixtures can be used on a daily basis. The hair will be left clean, although somewhat drier in some cases. Dryness is easily rectified by using a conditioner after washing, or switching to a dandruff shampoo with a built-in conditioner. (When using dandruff shampoos, avoid getting the shampoo in the eyes. The foaming ingredients can sting and cause tears and redness.)

Beware of coal tar–based dandruff shampoos if you have either white or gray hair. They may cause your hair to develop a muddy discolored stain.

When you shampoo on a daily basis, apply the shampoo, lather it in, let it sit according to the directions, and then rinse it out. This should take care of your dandruff problem. However, if you have an abnormal buildup of scale, you'll need to lather twice to obtain maximum efficacy.

You may notice after using your shampoo for a few weeks that it has lost some or all of its effectiveness. This is common. The body eventually develops a tolerance to different products, and you should change to a shampoo with different active ingredients.

If you are using a zinc pyrithione–based shampoo, and it doesn't have the same punch anymore, switch to one with selenium sulfide, and come at your dandruff from a different direction.

For African Americans, dandruff can be made worse by daily shampooing because regular and medicated shampoos tend to dry out the scalp. If this is the case, I recommend shampooing twice or three times a week with a dandruff shampoo. If that doesn't work to relieve symptoms, then see a dermatologist.

What the Doctor Will Do

When you consult a dermatologist for dandruff symptoms, the doctor will take a careful history and examination to determine that you do in fact have dandruff. A corticosteroid lotion may be prescribed to use after washing the hair. When applied to the scalp, this medication helps tone down dandruff. Oftentimes, people get their dandruff under control after just a few applications and can go back to shampooing with medicated dandruff shampoo. In some cases, however, they may still require corticosteroid treatment intermittently.

WHAT TO DO

- Wash your hair daily with your regular shampoo.
- If you can't wash daily, double your normal weekly frequency.
- For moderate to severe dandruff, switch to a specially formulated dandruff shampoo available in the pharmacy and use daily. Follow directions, lather once, and rinse out. For severe dandruff, perform the lather-rinse cycle twice.
- If hair becomes too dry from the constant washing, use a conditioner or switch to a shampoo with a built-in conditioner.
- For white or gray hair, avoid coal tar–based dandruff shampoos because they may stain your hair a muddy brown color.
- Switch to a shampoo with a different chemical formulation once you find your regular shampoo losing effectiveness.
- For severe dandruff that doesn't respond to frequent shampooing, consult a dermatologist.

DRY SKIN

Albert M. Kligman, M.D.

Dr. Kligman is professor of Dermatology at the University of Pennsylvania School of Medicine in Philadelphia, Pennsylvania

The symptoms of dry skin are unmistakable. The skin looks dry, and if you rub your finger over it, it is scaly, brittle, and rough. In moderate to severe cases of dry skin, the skin tends to itch, and constant scratching causes the skin to crack. This leads to pain, which can interfere with sleep. In the elderly, scratching is often complicated by infection. The cause of this vexing and common problem remains a mystery.

Dry skin is one of the unfortunate consequences of aging, because the skin cells just don't form correctly anymore. The dead cells shed from the surface tend to form clumps, which are visible as flakes and scales. This is a problem I experienced firsthand after I turned sixty-five.

Although the skin on my legs is dry, especially the lower portions, there are many measures that I now take in order to prevent dry skin from becoming a nuisance.

Treatment

Humidification is very important. When you take away moisture, things tend to dry out. In the winter, the worst thing you can do is turn up the heat; this lowers the relative humidity and allows the surface to dry out. House plants, furniture, and your skin are all adversely affected by low humidity in the air.

Instead of raising the thermostat, I lower it and open the windows in the house. Cold air has a higher relative humidity and is less drying. Of course, extremely cold, windy weather is to be avoided.

If you feel cold after opening the windows, put on warmer clothing. Avoid wool fabrics coming in direct contact with the skin because its rough texture tends to catch and move the skin scales, and this leads to itching and then scratching, setting up a vicious cycle that is difficult to break.

If it's not practical to keep your home cool, at least keep the heat turned down in your bedroom or purchase a humidifier.

In the summer months, avoid air-conditioning whenever possible. Once you go from a humid environment into a room with air-conditioning, the relative humidity is very low, and you'll lose water from your skin.

Dry skin is also precipitated year-round by frequent bathing in hot water. Over-bathing, in a tub especially, causes damage to the cell membranes, possibly by removing oil constituents. And when you use a soap that lathers up too much—a sign of high detergency—you're going to get into a lot of trouble because this damages the horny layer and forms tiny cracks and fissures in the skin.

When you use the tub, bathe less frequently and switch to a mild, gentle soap for personal hygiene. Use liquid soaps; they are milder than soap bars.

Don't put bath oil in your tub water because this increases the risk of slipping. Instead, take a soapless bath in warm water, and soak for 15 minutes to hydrate the skin. Then, dry yourself thoroughly, and seal in the moisture with a thin layer of petroleum jelly or a good moisturizing cream applied to your affected areas.

I have found the most effective way to treat dry skin is to use petroleum jelly on a daily basis. The gunkier the product the better. Most people hate this emollient because it's so messy to use, but it really does the best job of sealing in moisture and changing the surface of the skin. More than 90 percent of dry skin cases can be handled successfully with petroleum jelly alone.

A good trick for those who find greasiness objectionable is to apply petroleum jelly with a vigorous massage and then remove the excess with tissue. The portion that has entered the skin cannot be removed.

The jelly, a mixture of hydrocarbons and petroleum by-products, directly insinuates itself into the intercellular spaces of the horny layer of the skin, becoming a part of the skin, keeping it flexible and soft.

There's certainly nothing wrong with many (but not all) of the expensive lotions formulated for dry skin that you can buy at the pharmacy or department store. Use creams rather than lotions since these contain more oil, leaving more on the surface. These products work to ameliorate dry skin, but they're not as effective as petroleum jelly because they're mainly made of water. Once the water evaporates after the product is rubbed in, you're left with just a tiny bit of oil to coat your dry, flaking skin. And this includes the aloe-containing products as well; there is no proof of their efficacy in relieving dry skin symptoms.

Prevention

Prevention is the best treatment for dry skin, and those who have recurring winter dryness should start moisturizing the skin in November. I apply petroleum jelly at night, just before going to sleep. There is no need to grease yourself heavily with it. A little goes a long way. Rub it in gently and then use a tissue, and take off any excess.

A partner can be a great help in massaging in the jelly in difficult-to-reach areas.

This is a very simple, inexpensive, highly effective treatment. If you do this every night, you're not going to show any skin roughness. However, if you stop the applications, within two weeks dry skin symptoms will return.

WHAT TO DO

- Increase the relative humidity in your home by turning down the thermostat and opening windows. Use a humidifier if this isn't possible.

- Do not wear wool clothing that has direct skin contact. Wool fibers catch on scales and induce itching, which causes scratching. A vicious itch-scratch-itch-scratch cycle is set up.
- Bathe in warm water for at least 15 minutes and use a mild soap or no soap at all.
- Avoid frequent washing.
- Use the newer liquid soaps. They are milder than soap bars.
- Apply a thin film of petroleum jelly to affected areas each night. If this is too greasy, use a moisturizing cream recommended by your doctor. Effective brands include Moisturel and Lubriderm.

ECZEMA

James G. Marks, Jr., M.D.

Dr. Marks is professor of medicine, Division of Dermatology,
Pennsylvania State University, College of Medicine in Hershey, Pennsylvania

Eczema is a general term for many undiagnosed, noncontagious skin rashes and inflammatory reactions that are characterized by itching, redness, oozing, and blistering. These symptoms are variable and intermittent. For some, the affected skin often becomes thickened and discolored due to chronic scratching. For others, eczema is only episodic, responds well to different treatments, can be kept under control, and often vanishes, never to return.

Dermatologists refer to eczemas more specifically as dermatitis, an inflammation of the skin. There are different types of eczemas, some identified by causes, others by specific symptoms and location on the body. These include atopic dermatitis, seborrheic dermatitis, stasis dermatitis, and contact dermatitis, with its two subgroups, irritant and allergic dermatitis.

Atopic Dermatitis

Atopic dermatitis afflicts 5 percent of children, and can linger into adulthood. It usually starts after two months of age with a rash that affects the mouth and cheeks. Mild prescription hydrocortisone creams are often administered to relieve symptoms.

By five years of age, 90 percent of the children who will develop atopic eczema have already manifested its symptoms, which by this time include fierce itching and extremely dry skin, especially behind the knees and the creases in the elbows. Children often develop secondary bacterial infections because of their constant scratching, with the cracked skin providing a ready entry point for bacteria.

This infant and childhood form of eczema will usually fade for some years, only to reappear again in early adolescence. For the lucky majority, it will completely disappear by the late twenties, but for some, it lasts throughout life. It is uncommon for adults to develop atopic eczema without a prior history of eczema in childhood.

As with younger sufferers of atopic eczema, itching is the common complaint with adults. The upper back, face, shoulders, and the bends of the elbows and knees are affected. No one is sure why this form of eczema occurs, but we do know that it is associated with hay fever and asthma in one third of people who develop it, and in two thirds of their family members.

Treatment

Treatment of atopic eczema is difficult because there isn't one specific remedy that works for everyone. However, I have found that relief can be gained once itching and scratching is controlled. First, keep nails cut as short as possible and try your best to resist the urge to dig in and scratch.

Many people I treat get temporary relief with a milk compress. To make a milk compress, pour very cold milk onto a gauze pad or washcloth and leave it on the affected area for 3 minutes. Remove and reapply another wet cloth for 3 more minutes. Repeat the process several times throughout the day as needed.

A soak in a warm tub for 15–20 minutes also relieves the itch and helps restore skin moisture. When you get out of the tub, rub in moisturizing body oil to seal in the moisture.

Rolled oats (oatmeal) can also provide itch relief. Pour a cup of dry oatmeal into a sock and soak it in the water, or else pour 2 cups of oatmeal directly into your bath water. I don't know what the oats do exactly, but for many people it brings soothing, temporary relief.

If oats don't help, try using tar. There are several tar emollients available OTC that provide an anti-inflammatory effect when added to the bath water. Follow the directions on the label and soak in the tub for 15–20 minutes.

When washing or bathing, do not use harsh soaps. These dry out your already dry skin by removing the natural oils. Several good mild soaps or soap substitutes for personal hygiene are available OTC, as well as soapless cleansers.

Except for extremely mild cases, where an OTC 1% hydrocortisone cream may work, OTC antihistamines and cortisone creams are worthless for relieving the itch of atopic dermatitis. Save your money for the prescription-dosage medication that is really needed.

For severe cases, after applying post-bath moisturizing lotion, rub in a prescription topical steroid cream to help eliminate itching. Take a bath in the morning and again at night for maximum relief, repeating the oil-and-steroid-cream routine.

With a moderate to severe case, it usually takes a week or so to show results after beginning home treatment.

Prevention

There is a controversial and as yet unsubstantiated theory that atopic dermatitis may be prevented by having an infant avoid cow's milk, wheat, and eggs for the first six months of life. More research may lead to a definitive answer on this issue.

Seborrheic Dermatitis

Seborrheic dermatitis is a common, chronic, superficial, inflammatory process that affects the hairy regions of the body, especially the scalp, eyebrows, and face. Symptoms include red, scaly, and greasy skin patches.

In infants, this ailment is called cradle cap, and appears as patches of crusty skin. It usually fades after six to eight months. It's suspected that the eczema is caused by a yeast growing in a greasy, hairy area.

Treatment

To treat cradle cap effectively, rub either mineral oil or baby oil into the scalp at bedtime and leave it on overnight. The next day, wash the hair with a mild shampoo, dry the hair and brush. Repeat the treatment until cradle cap is eliminated. If it worsens, have the child seen by the pediatrician.

Seborrheic dermatitis vanishes shortly after infancy and can return at puberty as hormonal activity increases. In adults, red patches often appear in the scalp, accompanied by scaling and flaking that is actually an inflammatory form of dandruff. Scaly red patches may also appear on the hairline and on the nose, in the beard, sideburns, ear canals, and forehead.

Seborrheic dermatitis is easily treated in adults with antidandruff shampoos containing selenium sulfide or zinc pyrithione.

Shampoo twice a week with one of these shampoos, rubbing it in gently, allowing 5–10 minutes before rinsing. These shampoos have some harsh ingredients, and you may find your hair is a bit drier after use. If so, use a conditioner after shampooing.

After a few treatments you should notice relief. However, if the shampoo isn't working, or if the condition worsens, consult your dermatologist. A stronger shampoo can be prescribed, as well as a steroid lotion or gel that can be applied to the scalp and other affected areas.

Contact Dermatitis

Contact dermatitis, a common skin reaction manifested by skin redness and inflammation, is caused by coming into contact with a chemical to which you are allergic or which is irritating to your skin. There are two types: irritant and allergic dermatitis.

Skin damage is usually evident after contact, and symptoms of redness and itching generally develop eight to twelve hours later. Sometimes they may be delayed for four to seven days. The most common types and causes of allergic contact dermatitis include diaper rash, poison ivy, paraphenylenediamine (a dye used for the permanent coloring of hair), nickel (a common metal that 10 percent of the American female population is allergic to), rubber compounds (glues that bond the upper with the soles of shoes as a very common source), ethylenediamine (a preservative found in Mycolog cream, a common prescription drug used in the topical treatment of skin conditions).

Irritant contact dermatitis is caused by touching a substance that has a direct toxic effect on the skin. These include acids, solvents, and detergents. Reaction time depends on length of exposure and concentration of the irritant. Skin damage is evident immediately, or it may take several hours.

Treatment

To relieve symptoms of contact dermatitis, use wet compresses (see atopic dermatitis), keep your nails cut short, and avoid scratching as much as possible.

If you suspect that your allergy is to detergent, use rubber gloves when washing dishes. Get special cotton liners and wear them under the gloves to create an effective barrier against the rubber. Apply hand lotion several times a day to restore moisture.

If you are allergic to a particular chemical and must come in contact with it in the course of your work, wear protective clothing.

For moderate to severe contact dermatitis, or for chronic cases, contact your dermatologist. After a thorough examination, treatment will usually begin with steroidal creams and oral medication.

Stasis Eczema

Stasis eczema is a chronic disease of middle-aged and older adults that is caused by the pooling of blood in the lower legs.

With increased pressure and resulting capillary damage, fluid leaks out of the veins and causes eczema of the lower legs that is typified by red-brown patches and dry and itchy skin.

Treatment

Stasis dermatitis is best managed by wearing support hose. Standing should be restricted throughout the day and feet kept elevated when sitting. If you're significantly overweight, you should begin a weight-reduction program.

Cause for Concern

In severe cases, an ulceration of the lower leg can develop, and your dermatologist must be consulted. Total bed rest with the feet elevated is mandatory. Topical steroids will be prescribed, and wet compresses will be used to relieve any oozing or crusting.

What the Doctor Will Do

For cases of moderate to severe eczema, contact your dermatologist for help. After a thorough examination, systemic and topical steroids will most likely be prescribed, except for those people with high blood pressure and diabetes, who are given only topical steroid cream to use twice daily.

In time, with medication and regular treatment, eczema can be brought under control in most cases.

WHAT TO DO

To treat *atopic dermatitis:*
- Keep fingernails cut short.
- Use a milk compress and leave it on the affected area for 3 minutes. Repeat as needed.
- Soak in a warm tub for 15–20 minutes to increase the moisture content of the skin.
- Rub in moisturizing body oil or cream after bathing or whenever skin feels extra dry.
- Use a mild soap for bathing. For personal hygiene, use a soapless substitute available in the pharmacy.
- Use OTC antihistamines or hydrocortisone cream for itching relief.

To treat *seborrheic dermatitis,* an inflammation that affects the hairy regions of the body and appears as red, scaly, and greasy skin patches:
- Shampoo twice weekly with a dandruff shampoo containing selenium sulfide or zinc pyrithione; use a conditioner if hair becomes dry.

If treatment fails to relieve symptoms, contact your dermatologist for an examination.

To treat the rash and itching of allergic or irritant *contact dermatitis:*
- Eliminate sources of reaction, such as harsh chemicals and household cleansers.
- Wear protective clothing when handling irritants or allergens.
- For diaper rash, change diapers frequently, wash the groin area with a mild soap, and apply petroleum jelly.
- Apply a cool compress to the area.
- For mild cases, apply hydrocortisone cream to the area.

Contact your dermatologist if symptoms become more severe.

To treat *stasis eczema,* the red-brown, scaly patches that appear on the foot and lower extremity:
- Wear support hose.
- Restrict standing throughout the day and elevate the feet when possible.
- Start a weight-control program if overweight.

HIVES

Ivor Caro, M.D.

Dr. Caro is clinical associate professor of medicine (Dermatology), University of Washington School of Medicine in Seattle, Washington

Hives, or urticaria, are itchy, swollen, stinging, red patches or lumps that erupt suddenly on the body. They may develop a white center. Hives are caused by an allergic reaction to a substance, virus, insect bite, tension, or emotional stress. In more severe cases, called angioedema, there is swelling of the mucous membranes, eyelids, lips, and tongue.

Hives usually last for an hour or so, and may recur on and off for months. It is estimated that 20 percent of Americans will develop hives at least once, and many never know the underlying cause.

Hives can be divided into two major groups. *Acute hives* start suddenly, sometimes within minutes after exposure to the offending agent, and last for a short time. *Chronic hives* may develop suddenly or slowly and last much longer, remaining until the underlying cause is diagnosed and treated. The accepted dividing line between acute and chronic hives is six weeks. Chronic hives need to be treated by a physician.

The major cause of hives is a mild reaction to something you eat, touch, or even inhale. If you have had no previous problem with medicines or foods and develop hives out of the blue, it means that you may only now be allergic. You need to be careful about certain medications and foods.

Antibiotics are frequently the cause of hives, and penicillin is a classic cause. Even if you've taken it forty or fifty times in your lifetime without any problem, you can still develop hives quite suddenly from this drug.

Other common medicines can lead to hives. Aspirin is often a prime offender, as is the coating used on multivitamins and pill colorings.

Viral infections, flulike illnesses, and sore throats may cause hives, as can hepatitis, sinusitis, and mononucleosis.

People may develop hives after exposure to cold temperatures. Others will develop hives after a hot shower or bath. Bathe in tepid water instead. Inhaled house dust, pollen, flour, and dander from horses or cats are also prime hive triggers for some people. Avoidance is the best course here, coupled with prescription allergy medication from an allergist. In cases where extreme emotional anxiety or stress triggers hives, contact your physician. Counseling plus medication may be in order.

Insect bites and stings, not only from bees but sometimes from fleas, bedbugs, chiggers, and mosquitoes can also trigger hives.

Treatment

The best way to relieve the itching and swelling that come with hives is to take an OTC oral antihistamine such as Chlor-Trimeton or Benadryl. Children should be given liquid preparations. Although other home treatments for hives may provide temporary symptomatic relief, it is the antihistamine that is the mainstay of hive therapy. Be aware: most antihistamines will produce drowsiness, so follow package directions.

For practical purposes, these antihistamine medications are the same when it comes to hives, and they work fairly rapidly to reduce the accompanying redness, swelling, and itching.

Most topical anti-itch treatments available in the pharmacy do not work for hives. Hydrocortisone cream, which works well to relieve itching from insect bites, has no affect on hives. Avoid all OTC products labeled "topical anesthetic agents" or "topical antihistamines" because there is a risk of producing an allergic skin reaction.

For temporary relief of itching and swelling of small, localized hives, rub ice directly over the hives for several minutes, or take a cool shower. This slows down the release of itch-causing histamines into the bloodstream.

Soak in a tepid bath and add a special OTC oatmeal preparation such as Aveeno. This will temporarily soothe and cool the skin.

Cause for Concern

If you develop hives while you are on medication for some other condition, consult with your physician immediately. Don't continue with the medication because it may be what is causing the hives, and the next dose may bring on severe swelling of the lips and throat, and interfere with breathing and swallowing. It may also lead to anaphylactic shock, a life-threatening reaction that causes severe swelling, dizziness, and even loss of consciousness. The doctor will change your prescription.

Adverse reaction to certain foods is another cause of hives. If you develop hives that settle down but recur twenty-four, forty-eight, or seventy-two hours later, carefully review the foods you have eaten within that period. It may take painstaking detective work to find the culprit, but it is needed. Shellfish, dairy products, nuts, pork, strawberries, chocolate, tomatoes, and oranges are all prime suspects.

If you develop more severe symptoms after eating—swelling of the lips, tightness in the chest, difficulty in swallowing, or wheezing—you need to eliminate that food from your diet forever.

If you develop a big hive after being stung by a bee or other biting insect, contact your doctor. You may be advised to carry a prescription anaphylaxis emergency kit with you at all times. There are two types of kits available. EpiPen has a spring-released needle, while the Ana-Kit comes with a syringe. The doctor will show you how to use the device. Both work by injecting a dose of the stimulant epinephrine, which counteracts the reaction and prevents swelling.

What the Doctor Will Do

If home treatment fails, contact your family physician. The doctor will take a good oral history, going over diet, medication, and any recent sickness. If the hives are chronic, special lab studies may be performed. If the hives are itching terribly, a powerful antihistamine may be injected and can bring rapid relief. Cortisone may also be injected or else oral cortisone may be prescribed.

If more severe symptoms develop such as swollen lips and tongue, wheezing, or dizziness, seek medical attention.

WHAT TO DO

- Take an oral antihistamine tablet such as Chlor-Trimeton or Benadryl. Children need to take a liquid preparation.
- Apply ice directly to the hives when they are not too widespread.
- Take a cool shower.
- Soak in a tepid bath and add an oatmeal preparation to that water such as Aveeno that is available without prescription at the pharmacy.
- Medications such as antibiotics and aspirin, and foods such as shellfish, chocolate, and dairy products may cause hives. Consult your physician if medication is a hive trigger and eliminate hive-causing foods from the diet.

INSECT BITES AND STINGS: BEES AND SPIDERS

John B. McCabe, M.D.

Dr. McCabe is professor and chairman, Department of Emergency Medicine at the State University of New York Health Service Center in Syracuse, New York

Biting, stinging insects such as bees, wasps, yellow jackets, and spiders are all around us, and once you invade their territory, you may come away with a sting or a bite that ranges from mild to dangerous.

Bee Stings

Bee stings are usually temporary, painful nuisances, which cause local skin reactions that clear up in a matter of hours.

The female honeybee has a short black body with yellow and black markings. When this bee attacks a human, its hook-shaped barbed stinger detaches along with internal organs and remains lodged in the skin. The bee dies soon after. To prevent injection of more venom into the skin from this venom sac, it must be removed immediately.

Don't try to pull the stinger out with your fingers or tweezers because this will only cause more venom to be released. Instead, scrape your fingernail, a knife blade, or credit card quickly over the stinger and attempt to flick it out.

Wasps and yellow jackets have stingers that remain intact and can be used for multiple stings. So, if you're attacked once by them, leave the area immediately to avoid another sting.

Treatment

Bees are scavengers who often go through garbage in the course of their travels, so whenever I'm stung, I'll immediately wash the area with soap and water to prevent any bacterial infection from starting. I then put something very cold on the sting to reduce pain and swelling. My first choice is an ice cube, but if that's not available, I'll use cold, running water instead. Even a cold can of soda applied to the area will work. For maximum relief, keep the sting area cold for at least a half hour.

Even with the application of cold, there may be significant pain for an hour or so. If the pain, swelling, and itch still persist, take an antihistamine such as diphenhydramine (Benadryl), available OTC in any pharmacy. Follow label directions for dosage. Two aspirin tablets can also relieve swelling and itching.

Prevention

Bees and wasps are both attracted to bright colors, cooking odors, and perfume. If you're going to be in their territory
- Wear neutral colored clothing.
- Avoid strong perfume, scented soap, after-shave, and hair spray.
- When you're in the garden or out for a walk in the field, wear shoes to avoid being stung on the feet.

- Make sure garbage pails are tightly covered and that all holes are patched in house screens.

Cause for Concern

An estimated 2 million Americans are extremely allergic to bee venom, and for these hypersensitive individuals, stings can bring on anaphylactic shock, a severe reaction that begins within a matter of minutes. Symptoms may include nausea; bronchospasm with its wheezing and difficulty in breathing; cool, clammy, and pale skin; rapid pulse; diarrhea; cramps; extreme thirst; dizziness; loss of consciousness; and, if not treated immediately, death.

Another secondary sign of this allergic reaction is swelling in the back of the throat, which leads to difficulty in both breathing and swallowing. Contact your physician or hospital Emergency Department immediately for treatment. Fifteen to twenty Americans die each year from bee stings, mostly from these severe allergic reactions. However, treatment is very effective, and fatalities can be prevented once emergency measures are started.

In the Emergency Department, the hormone epinephrine will be injected to improve breathing. Once you become stabilized, be prepared to contact an allergist for extensive testing, and possibly to start a course of desensitization injections that will be given year-round. You may also need to carry with you at all times a special emergency kit, containing a syringe and epinephrine. When stung by a bee, inject yourself with the epinephrine to counteract the venom and then head to the Emergency Department for further treatment.

Spider Bites

Of the many spiders in North America, household spiders are generally harmless to humans, but the brown recluse spider and the black widow are both potentially dangerous because of their venom.

Treatment

The bite of the household spider can cause some redness of the skin and minor infection, but nothing more. This particular spider bite is best treated by cleansing the area with soap and water.

Cause for Concern

The black widow spider is easily recognized by the characteristic red hourglass mark on its abdomen. Although its bite is often painless, the venom produced by the female black widow causes a powerful systemic reaction that often mimics appendicitis. Nausea, vomiting, and stomach pain and spasms are the major symptoms, and you may be sick for several days. Bed rest is imperative, but the venom results in a self-limiting illness that will resolve by itself.

In severe cases involving the very young, the very old, or people who develop malaise, joint pain, or high fever, a special serum may be administered in the Emergency Department. This serum is an effective spider-poison antidote, but in many cases people have a delayed reaction to it and develop "serum sickness" that may sometimes make them even sicker.

The venom of the brown recluse spider, also known as a fiddler or violin spider because of the fiddlelike marking on its back, is powerful. Not only is this spider reclusive, but most people aren't even aware that they've been bitten. Initially you may itch and have a small puncture from the spider's bite, but within a few hours local skin reactions may appear, including minor pain, swelling, and discoloration around the bite where the venom was injected. If this happens, go to your doctor or hospital Emergency Department.

If left untreated, over the next few days the skin will develop ulcers and slowly start to die. Disfiguring scars are not uncommon. Before going to the Emergency Department or doctor, apply ice or a cold compress to reduce the swelling. The doctor will provide pain medication and antibiotics.

When there's a break in the skin, whether from a bee sting or a spider bite, you're at risk of tetanus infection. Tetanus is an infection of the nervous system caused by a dirt-borne bacterium, *Clostridium tetani,* that enters open wounds. It eventually affects muscle contraction. Although there is not much tetanus in this country because of widespread immunization, anytime you are bitten or stung, be sure that your tetanus immunization is up to date.

If you're not sure when you had your last tetanus shot, the doctor will give you a booster shot that will last for ten years.

WHAT TO DO

- Apply ice or cold running water to the sting for 30 minutes.
- If pain persists, take an antihistamine tablet containing diphenhydramine, or take 2 aspirin tablets.
- If you develop any abnormal swelling at the bite site, feel dizzy, or have difficulty breathing, contact your physician, go to the nearest Emergency Department for treatment, or call 911 for help.
- If bitten by a black widow spider, rest in bed to get through the cramps and nausea caused by the bite. In severe cases, muscle relaxants may be administered. If pain continues, spider serum is given. Side effects are common.
- When bitten by a brown recluse spider, apply ice or a cold compress to the site to reduce swelling. Contact your physician immediately.

JOCK ITCH
Lowell A. Goldsmith, M.D.

Dr. Goldsmith is the James H. Sterner Professor and chairman, Department of Dermatology, University of Rochester School of Medicine and Dentistry in Rochester, New York

Jock itch, or tinea cruris, is a common fungal infection that affects the groin area of men and, in rare cases, women. It is contagious. Typical symptoms include itchy, red scaly patches on the groin, thighs, and buttocks. Pus-filled blisters can also develop.

People who exercise regularly and wear

an athletic supporter (jock strap) are susceptible to jock itch if they don't bathe after exercise. Also, people who wear tight, constricting clothing or jockey underpants made of synthetics, or wear clothing for extended periods of time, are also very susceptible to the jock itch fungus.

In addition to poorly ventilated clothing, friction is also a cause of jock itch. If you are overweight and your thighs rub against each other when you walk or exert yourself, you're a probable candidate for jock itch.

If you sit in a car or airplane seat for extended periods of time, you lose the ability to evaporate sweat from the groin area, and therefore create a prime breeding ground for the jock itch fungus.

Moisture seems to be a critical factor with jock itch. Since we all wear clothing for most of the day, the groin is usually dark and warm. But once it becomes moist, two types of microscopic fungi that ordinarily live on the skin, dermatophytes and candidae, can multiply and cause trouble. Jock itch is especially prevalent in warm, humid climates and during the summer months.

If jock itch isn't treated, the infection tends to become chronic and can quickly spread to the buttocks and trunk.

Treatment

Proper hygiene, antifungal medication, and the elimination of the warm, moist environment of the groin are essential in the treatment of jock itch.

Wash the affected area gently with soap and water. Rinse the soap completely from the area to prevent irritation and dry yourself thoroughly. Twice daily apply a light layer of clotrimazole (Lotrimin), a generic antifungal compound now available OTC. This medication works against both the candida and dermatophyte fungus. You should start seeing results in three to five days. Continue to use the medication for another three to five days after the rash has cleared up. When the rash is nearly healed, use cornstarch-free powder (Zeasorb AF) after bathing to keep the groin region moisture-free.

In addition, other steps should be taken. After swimming, don't sit around in a wet suit. Air is a good deterrent, so to aid in ventilation, wear loose, cotton boxer-type underwear and change it daily. Be sure to wear clean athletic clothes and underwear for workouts. If you're overweight and perspire heavily, it's advisable to lose weight.

If these conservative steps fail to clear the jock itch or prevent recurrence, contact a dermatologist.

What the Doctor Will Do

After taking your case history, the doctor will use a scalpel to scrape off scales or pustules and examine them under the microscope in order to render a precise diagnosis.

It's important during the doctor's exam to remove your socks to have your feet checked. Toes and feet are potential sites for the dermatophyte fungus.

Once a diagnosis of jock itch has been confirmed, the doctor may prescribe oral antifungal medication, generally ketoconazole, or griseofulvin if it's a dermatophyte. This will be taken for two weeks and then another evaluation will be given. There is usually no need to continue the medication after this time.

WHAT TO DO

- Gently wash the affected areas with soap and water.
- Apply clotrimazole cream twice daily.
- Apply antifungal powder to the area to keep it dry.
- Wear cotton boxer-type underwear and change daily.
- If you are overweight and perspire heavily, lose weight.
- Contact your dermatologist if these conservative steps fail to relieve symptoms.

LICE

Deborah G. Haynes, M.D.

Dr. Haynes is clinical assistant professor, University of Kansas School of Medicine, Wichita, Kansas

Lice are flat, wingless parasites the size of a pinhead that live on the body. In order to survive, the lice pierce the skin and feed off human blood. This causes their bodies to darken and at the same time leads to intense itching and skin inflammation on the victim.

Three types of lice affect humans—head lice, pubic lice, and body lice. All can be eradicated when they are treated with an insecticide, and all clothing and home furnishings are thoroughly cleaned.

Female lice lay approximately six eggs daily. These eggs, or nits, are tiny translucent specks that look like dandruff and cling firmly to hair shafts. They hatch in eight to ten days and reach maturity in eighteen days. They may remain viable for three weeks. If lice are not treated with an insecticidal shampoo, cream, or lotion, they can spread quickly, infesting anyone who comes in close contact.

Head Lice

Head lice are the most common type, especially among schoolchildren. Children often wear each other's hats, use one another's combs, or may share naptime pillows.

Good personal hygiene habits don't protect against head lice infestation. My children are scrupulously clean, but they have still come home from school with head lice. One time, before the infestation was finally stopped, more than fifty of their classmates also had lice. It is not uncommon for schools and summer camps to close temporarily to stop an infestation.

Typical symptoms of head lice include itching of the scalp and neck, red bite marks, and tiny, white-colored nits on the hair. In some severe cases, the lymph glands at the back of the neck may swell.

Treatment

There is only one effective way to kill head lice, and that is by using a specially formulated insecticide shampoo. Three shampoos available OTC are A-200, R & C, and Rid. Of the available insecticides, they are the least toxic to humans.

There are also prescription medicines available for lice: lindane (Kwell), permethrin (Nix), and malathion (Ovide). Lindane and pyrethrin are equally effective. Malathion has a high level of egg-killing activity. Follow directions carefully on the label for all insecticides. In most cases, a onetime application will kill the lice. After rinsing the shampoo out of your hair, dry thoroughly. Wash the towel in hot water and detergent and dry in a dryer set on the hot cycle before using it again.

Although antilice shampoos stop initial infestation, they do not kill all of the unhatched nits. To accomplish this, illuminate the hair in natural sunlight or examine closely with a flashlight. Use a pair of fine tweezers to remove the nits from the hair shafts. This is a time-consuming task, but *all* nits must be removed or reinfestation will soon occur.

For nit removal, begin in one part of the scalp with a small amount of hair, and then systematically move row by narrow row (strand by strand in some cases) and pick off the nits. If you use the fine-toothed nit comb supplied with most louse shampoo kits, dip it first in hot vinegar. The vinegar helps to loosen the nits from the hair follicles. Repeatedly run the dampened comb through the hair from the scalp outward. Check the comb for nits after each pass and remove them before dipping it again in the vinegar. For the next ten days, continue to check the hair daily. Shampoo again in one week to kill any newly hatched lice that may have been missed.

Soak all combs and brushes for several hours in a lice shampoo solution and then wash them thoroughly.

A close haircut will not remove all head lice because they can still cling to any remaining hair.

All bedding that an infested person used must be either dry-cleaned or washed in hot soapy water and dried at a high temperature to kill the lice. In addition, vacuum all mattresses, rugs, upholstered couches, and chairs.

If an item cannot be washed or dry-cleaned, put it into a plastic bag with an airtight seal for two to three weeks. When deprived of human blood, the lice will die.

To prevent further infestation, immediately notify anyone who may have had close physical contact with the affected person, so they can be examined.

Pubic Lice

Pubic lice, also known as "crabs" because they resemble them, are tiny wingless parasites that attach securely to hair follicles in the pubic area and feed off human blood. This causes a maddening, unrelenting itch. In some cases, this infestation can lead to a blue-gray discoloration of the skin that looks like a bruise. This is a result of bleeding caused by the blood-sucking lice. They are spread through sexual contact or contact with lice-infested bedding or clothing.

Treatment

Pubic lice are effectively eradicated with OTC antilice preparations A-200, R & C, or Rid, the same ones used for head lice. Apply the insecticide according to directions. Use tweezers to remove all nits, the tiny, white eggs of lice.

Dry-clean or wash all clothing and bedding in hot soapy water and dry in a dryer set on the hot cycle.

Contact all sexual partners so they may be checked and treated for lice as well.

Body Lice

Cases of body-lice infestation are rarely seen in this country. They are most common in overcrowded urban areas with little or no sanitation.

Body lice live in the seams of soiled clothing and come out to feed off human blood, causing intense itching. Body lice are eradicated with an OTC insecticide lotion such as RID or A-200. Wash all clothing in hot soapy water and dry in a dryer on the hot cycle.

One application of insecticide is generally enough to kill all head, pubic, and body lice.

What the Doctor Will Do

If the OTC medicated shampoo, lotion, or cream fails to eradicate the lice, or if the lice infest the eyebrows or eyelashes, contact your physician. After close examination and diagnosis, lice will be carefully removed from the eye area by the doctor. The doctor may prescribe either lindane or pyrethrin, two effective prescription insecticides.

WHAT TO DO

- Apply a specially formulated OTC insecticide shampoo, lotion, or cream according to directions, or obtain prescription medication from your physician.
- Use a pair of tweezers or a special nit comb to get rid of the translucent nits (lice eggs) that are cemented to hair follicles.
- Reapply the insecticide in one week to kill any newly hatched lice.
- Dry-clean or wash all bedding the infested person used in hot, soapy water and then dry with hot heat to make sure all lice are killed.
- Vacuum all mattresses, rugs, upholstered couches, and chairs that an infested person may have come in contact with.
- To prevent further infestation, don't share any combs, brushes, hats, or scarves. Notify anyone who may have had close physical contact with the affected person so they can be examined.
- Contact your physician if you have lice in the eyebrows or eyelashes, or if the insecticide fails to eradicate the lice.

POISON IVY

William P. Jordan, M.D.

Dr. Jordan is director of Dermatology Research at a private contract laboratory in Richmond, Virginia

The red, itching skin eruptions we call poison ivy occur when a foreign substance—the poison ivy resin—is totally rejected by the body. This allergic reaction takes two to three weeks to resolve even with immediate attention to the problem.

Poison ivy and its relatives, poison oak and poison sumac, can grow as a plant, a vine, or a bush. The three leaflets are shiny or dull, up to 5 inches in length, with edges that can be jagged or smooth. Green in the summertime, the leaves turn yellow or pinkish-red in the autumn. Although it changes color with the seasons, the plant remains poisonous year-round.

If you've never been exposed—and you have the tendency to develop an allergy to the plant's oil—the immunological development that will initially sensitize you and make you allergic to the oil takes about seven to twenty days after your first brush with the plant. All subsequent exposures to poison ivy are rapid and bring on reactions eight to ninety-six hours later.

Once contact is made with the plant, an intense red, itchy rash soon develops on your skin. The shape of this itchy rash is directly related to the way you rubbed against the plant. Scattered patches of rash on the skin result from streaking the poison ivy resin with your hands.

The oil is easily transmitted at any time of the year on the fur of cats and dogs, and can adhere to shoes and clothing as well. Just touch the contaminated animals or clothing, and you'll develop a reaction.

If you inhale the fumes from a burning poison ivy plant, the result can be inflamed lungs, wheezing, and shortness of breath. Each year, more than 30 percent of California forest firefighters have to come off the lines because of reactions to inhaled poison ivy.

Treatment

If I think I've been exposed to poison ivy, I wash the affected area as soon as possible with cold running water. A thorough shower is also a good idea. This helps float some of the plant resin off the skin and keeps it from penetrating. Don't use soap or rubbing alcohol. These only help spread the resin.

Most OTC poison ivy remedies are ineffective for moderate to substantial cases of the rash. However, those that claim to offer relief of the terrible itch that accompanies poison ivy are useful if they have lidocaine or pramoxine HCL.

Once the rash has developed, OTC oral antihistamines may offer temporary relief from itching. If the case is very mild, I find that .5 percent hydrocortisone cream applied six to ten times daily works well for temporary relief of itching. Still, it pales next to the strength of poison ivy. Even the new, higher strength 1 percent hydrocortisone creams don't offer complete relief.

As the rash becomes more pronounced, starts to blister, and begins to ooze a clear fluid, use calamine lotion every three to four hours to dry the weeping. Apply the lotion to a clean cloth and gently pat the affected area.

Prevention

- The best way to prevent poison ivy is to know what it looks like and avoid it at all times.
- If you have to work or play in an area where you know it grows, wear long pants and a long-sleeved shirt, socks, even gloves.
- For more protection, there are now OTC lotions to put on exposed skin surfaces before you go outside. These products—Stokkogard is probably the best —form an effective barrier that reduce the penetration of any poison ivy oil.

What the Doctor Will Do

Even with these treatments, you won't cure poison ivy. By and large, you can't slow its course without prescription drugs, such as a powerful topical steroid or oral prednisone.

If your poison ivy symptoms are moderate to severe, consult with a physician who knows how to treat the ailment. Prednisone, a synthetic corticosteroid used to combat allergic conditions, should be prescribed. The tablets are taken for two weeks and have virtually no side effects because of the short treatment duration.

Prednisone is a miracle worker if prescribed effectively, but it's often not done well. In some cases a flare-up of poison ivy may occur if you come off the medication too early.

WHAT TO DO

- Wash yourself with cold running water to remove the sap as soon as you think you have been exposed.

For mild cases with a few localized areas of redness, itching, or pustules:
- Rub a 1 percent concentration of hydrocortisone cream six to eight times daily on the affected areas.
- Use calamine lotion every three or four hours to dry any weeping or oozing.

For moderate to severe cases of poison ivy typified by extensive red patches of skin, severe itching, and blistering, contact a dermatologist for drug therapy.

PSORIASIS

Nicholas J. Lowe, M.D.

Dr. Lowe is a clinical professor of Dermatology at the UCLA School of Medicine, and director of The Southern California Dermatology and Psoriasis Center in Santa Monica, California

Psoriasis is a chronic skin disorder typified by plaques, distinct patches of dry, reddened, inflamed skin that have a silvery scalelike appearance. Plaques are frequently found on the elbow creases, on the knees, and on the scalp. They may remain localized, or may spread to larger areas of the skin, including the toenails and fingernails. These plaques can develop into a form of arthritis just as severe as the rheumatoid type. Itching is a problem for about 30 percent of people with psoriasis.

In many cases, the skin becomes cracked, painful, and ultimately disfigured. Once it develops on the hands and feet, it can become disabling. Some people are unable to work because of it.

Psoriasis may be confused with seborrheic dermatitis (see page 188), atopic eczema (see page 186), or, when it affects infants, with diaper rash (see diaper rash in contact dermatitis section, page 188). Certain skin cancers may also look like psoriasis. For this reason, it's important to see a dermatologist, who will make the correct diagnosis and prescribe the proper course of treatment.

There are several things that can trigger psoriasis or worsen symptoms. These include sore throat infection, alcohol, obesity, stress, anxiety, certain medications and drugs, and damage to the skin through scrapes, cuts, or sunburn. Contrary to popular belief, there is no link between diet and psoriasis.

Treatment

To minimize the effects of psoriasis, sunbathing offers some benefit. Proceed cautiously, basking on a daily basis for 30 minutes to an hour. About 80 percent of people with psoriasis will see improvement after about three to six weeks. A half hour before sunbathing, apply sunscreen with SPF 15 (sun protection factor) on *nonpsoriasis* skin to protect against developing sunburn, which will aggravate psoriasis. Many people find psoriasis relief by vacationing in a sunny climate. Remission can last for long periods after such a trip.

Use plenty of moisturizers on your skin. However, avoid lanolin-based moisturizers if you are allergic to lanolin. Petroleum jelly and lactic acid–based moisturizers made by reputable companies keep the skin moist when used regularly, and can provide relief. Purchase the big 1-pound jars of petroleum jelly. When you get out of the bath, towel off slightly, and then rub in the jelly to trap the moisture to the skin.

Creams and ointments available OTC that contain salicylic acid help to soften and remove scales. OTC coal-tar gels and oils can also slow down the rate that the skin cells are produced, and thus improve psoriasis. Follow the instructions carefully when using a coal-tar preparation, because tars can react with sunlight and cause a bad sunburn.

Special bath solutions also may offer symptomatic relief of psoriasis. These mixtures contain either oatmeal, various oils, or coal tar. If you are allergic to tar, switch to another product. Follow instructions on the packages. Soak for 15 minutes in the tub, and this will help both your skin and your mood.

For psoriasis plaques in the scalp, a special softening gel that contains salicylic acid is available OTC. Apply it to the scalp at night according to the instructions, and then wash it out in the morning with a medicated dandruff shampoo such as Head and Shoulders.

When combing your hair, don't comb too vigorously. Anytime you scratch or scrape the scalp with a comb or brush, you increase the risk of having the psoriasis come back worse than before.

Try to avoid scratching the itch. If you feel like scratching, reach for your moisturizer and rub it on, or else rub on the medicated prescription cream your physician has given you. If you itch frequently, take an OTC antihistamine tablet at night.

If you are taking lithium for depression, it can adversely affect psoriasis. Contact your internist or psychiatrist to make sure it won't make your psoriasis worse. If stress makes your psoriasis worse, take effective steps to reduce your stress levels. You may want to avoid caffeine or similar stimulant drugs, which can make you more nervous. To this end, try stress reduction exercises such as yoga, biofeedback, or meditation. In many cases, even self-hypnosis can work wonders. You can learn the techniques for all of these exercises from books or audiotapes by professional instructors.

If psoriasis doesn't respond to various home measures, find a dermatologist who's used to treating psoriasis. For a referral in your area, contact the National Psoriasis Foundation, 6442 SW Beaverton Highway, Suite 201, Portland, Oregon 97221; 503-297-1545.

What the Doctor Will Do

The doctor will go into your complete medical and family history, and look for underlying causes that may be triggering psoriasis.

Many effective prescription medications should control psoriasis in most cases. By working with the doctor, you can alleviate many of your symptoms, sometimes for years.

Several topical creams, some cortisone-based, some containing coal tar or salicylic acid, and newer drugs with vitamin D structures show promise in promoting symptomatic relief. When used under a doctor's guidance, results usually come within weeks, sometimes sooner.

Once psoriasis improves or clears, treatment is usually stopped until the next episode. For some, maintenance dosages of medication are continued, even when psoriasis is gone.

I successfully treat many patients in the office with ultraviolet light therapy called PUV-A. The patient takes a Psoralen pill and then UV-A is shone onto the skin by a special machine. Besides improving the existing condition, this treatment prevents new psoriasis in other areas of the body.

If we apply too much UV-A, there may be a slightly increased risk of skin cancer in later years, both squamous cell and basal cell cancers. However, if used correctly, PUV-A is a very good treatment, with few if any internal side effects.

After a course of successful treatment, counseling by the doctor becomes especially important. People will often start wondering, "What if it comes back?" They can actually worry themselves right back into a recurrence. The doctor should reassure them that the psoriasis may come back, but that even if it does, treatment will stop it once again.

WHAT TO DO

- Apply a sunscreen 30 minutes before going outside. Sunbathe up to an hour but avoid sunburn, which will aggravate psoriasis.
- Apply a thin layer of skin moisturizer such as petroleum jelly, especially after bathing. Be wary of any coal-tar preparation, because it may cause skin irritation when exposed to the sun.

- Soak in the tub with a commercial tar or oatmeal preparation available at the pharmacy. Avoid tar if you are allergic to it.
- For psoriasis of the scalp, apply an OTC softening gel at night and shampoo it out the next morning with a medicated dandruff shampoo.
- To relieve the stress or tension that aggravates psoriasis, try yoga, meditation, biofeedback, or self-hypnosis.
- For moderate to severe cases of psoriasis, or if home remedies don't work to control psoriasis, contact a dermatologist who's had success treating the ailment.

RAZOR BURN

Richard B. Odom, M.D.

Dr. Odom is clinical professor of Dermatology and associate chairman of the Department of Dermatology at the University of California at San Francisco

Razor burn is a temporary skin irritation caused by shaving. The underlying causes may be a skin disorder such as eczema (see Eczema, page 186), ingrown hairs, or extreme skin dehydration brought on by either living in an overheated house or outdoor exposure to cold and wind. However, the most common cause of razor burn is improper preparation of the beard for shaving.

Treatment

If you nick the skin while shaving, use a styptic pencil, available at any pharmacy, to stop blood flow from these minor cuts. These pencils contain coagulants that control the bleeding immediately. If you don't have a styptic pencil available, take a tissue, double it over, place it directly on the cut, and apply pressure.

Ingrown beard hairs, easily recognized by the little red bumps on the neck and face, are the result of daily shaving and will cause minor razor burn every time you shave over them. Known as "razor bumps," they develop when the hair, cut sharply by a razor, bends over and starts growing back into the skin.

Razor bumps are a major problem for black men, because their naturally curly and coarse beard hairs hook back into the skin. The condition becomes extremely painful whenever these bumps are shaved over. Not only will they bleed when cut, but regular shaving will cause permanent scar tissue to develop. For men with severe razor bumps, there is no good solution, and I recommend that they stop shaving and grow a beard. For men who cannot grow a beard because of job restraints or personal preference, the individual ingrown hairs must be lifted out prior to shaving. To lift out an ingrown hair, stand in front of a mirror, take a sterilized straight pin, gently open the skin with the pin, and flick out the hair. Gently plucking this hair with tweezers may stop an immediate problem, but it doesn't offer a permanent solution because another hair soon grows in the hair follicle.

If razor bumps continue to be a problem, try a chemical depilatory available in any pharmacy. Depilatories work by chemically causing the hair to detach at the skin surface. In addition to its strong odor, the major drawback to a depilatory is the alkaline chemicals in the product, which may cause severe skin irritation if used more than every other day. If skin irritation does result, discontinue its use.

Prevention

- Soften the beard with moist heat. Wash your face with hot water or apply a hot, damp washcloth and keep it there for a minute or so, or shave in the shower.
- Use a gel foam specifically designed for sensitive skin. These have more lubricants to soften the beard and decrease razor friction. Let the foam sit for at least 2 minutes before shaving.
- Experiment with different kinds of razors, such as electric, disposable cartridge, double-edged blades, or disposables.
- Keep an electric razor on the medium setting. There is no evidence electric razors offer closer shaves, or are less likely to cause razor burn.
- If you're susceptible to razor burn, change your blade daily.
- Shave by following the grain of your beard.
- Pull your razor downward with the flow of your beard on your cheeks and chin, and pull upward on your neck. Shaving against the grain leads to razor burn.
- Don't stretch the skin during shaving. It may cause facial hair to curve and grow

downward, leading to razor burn and irritation.
- When finished shaving, rinse the face with warm water, then splash on cool water to hydrate the face.
- If your skin is sensitive, avoid all alcohol after-shaves and use aloe-based lotions instead.

What the Doctor Will Do

For men who regularly develop irritation from shaving, a visit to the dermatologist is in order. After a careful examination, the doctor may recommend a topical cortisone lotion to be applied after shaving in order to reduce inflammation. This should take care of most cases of razor irritation.

WHAT TO DO

- Moisten the beard with plenty of hot water or place a damp, hot washcloth on the face for 2 minutes. In lieu of this, shave in the shower at the completion of bathing.
- Use a shaving cream formulated for sensitive skin. Leave it on the skin for 2 minutes prior to shaving.
- Try different types of shaving devices to find which works best for your skin.
- Change your razor after each shave if your skin is particularly sensitive.
- Shave with the grain of your beard. Pull gently down on the face and chin, and pull upward on the neck.
- Don't pull the skin taut as you shave or shave back and cross against the beard. This often leads to ingrown hairs.
- Splash cool water on your face after

shaving to hydrate the skin. If you use an after-shave, make sure it's aloe-based.

- If you develop razor bumps or ingrown hairs from shaving, use a sterilized pin to flick each hair out of its follicle before shaving.

- If you must be clean shaven and razor bumps are a problem, use a depilatory instead of a razor.

- If shaving causes razor burn regularly, consult with a dermatologist for further treatment.

SUNBURN

Thomas P. Nigra, M.D.

Dr. Nigra is chairman of the Department of Dermatology, Washington Hospital Center, and clinical professor of Dermatology, George Washington University Medical School in Washington, D.C.

You're at the beach or on the golf course trying to break 90, when all of a sudden you realize you've been out in the sun too long. The result is sunburn, caused when the ultraviolet rays penetrate the skin and damage the underlying tissue. The specific rays responsible are most prevalent from 10 A.M. to 3 P.M. during the summer months. You can't get sunburned before 9 A.M. or after 5 P.M. because the sun's rays angle differently.

Sunburn pain can be bad enough, but now there is incontrovertible evidence that the sun can also cause serious, long-term damage to the skin. Frequent low-intensity sun exposure is a factor in the later development of nonmelanoma skin cancers: squamous cell skin cancer, as well as basal cell skin cancer, both of which are curable but can be disfiguring.

The real danger, however, is malignant melanoma, a potentially fatal form of skin cancer that is now linked to serious cases of sunburn, particularly repeated episodes during youth. Melanomas are now responsible for over 6,000 deaths annually in this country.

Melanoma arises around pigmented areas of the skin, such as moles or freckles. It typically occurs after the age of forty and develops as a very dark brown or black mole, usually with a notched pattern and red and white coloring within. Know which moles are normal for you, and you will notice what has become abnormal.

For early detection, use this ABCD system to help locate a cancer on your body. Check your entire body, from the top of your head to the soles of your feet.

A stands for asymmetry, an irregularity of shape. Draw a line through the mole's center, and there will not be two equally matching halves. A noncancerous mole is round and symmetrical.

B is for irregular border. Benign growths have very regular margins. Cancerous lesions have jagged edges.

C is for color. Cancerous lesions will have many colors, from tan and brown to black, often with pink mixed in with red and white. Benign growths usually are one color overall and flat.

D is for diameter. If the growth measures more than a quarter inch across, it may be dangerous.

If you have any suspicion of melanoma, contact your dermatologist *immediately.*

There are three distinct degrees of sunburn: first-degree burn, which causes the skin to turn bright red; second-degree burn, characterized by the appearance of blisters; and third-degree burn, characterized by the skin turning black or white, and often by the absence of any pain. Second-degree sunburn is quite rare and third-degree burn, caused by prolonged, high-intensity sun exposure, is extremely rare.

By far, the most common type of sunburn is first-degree, the painful garden variety burn that you get from staying unprotected out in the sun too long. Just because your skin hasn't turned pink, don't think you haven't been burned. A sunburn is most evident anywhere from six to twenty-four hours after you've been exposed.

Contrary to popular belief, the idea of a "protective tan" is misleading. A tan will protect you from sunburn, but it can't prevent damage caused by repeated ultraviolet ray exposure, which breaks down the elastic fibers of the skin. Over time, this ultimately leads to wrinkling, sagging, damaged blood vessels, as well as an increased risk of skin cancer.

Prevention

There are now a variety of sun-shielding agents on the market in oil, lotion, or cream form that do a great job in protecting you from overexposure. Most of them are easy to apply and not very visible on the skin. Follow the directions for application to obtain maximum protection. Research has shown that most people underapply sunscreen, thereby reducing their protection, sometimes dramatically.

All sunscreens now come with sun protection factor (SPF) ratings, generally reliable indicators given in numbers from 2 up to 45 SPF. These ratings let you know the number of times longer you can stay in the sun before burning after using the sunscreen than if you had used nothing. For example, if you would normally start to turn pink in 20 minutes, then a sunscreen with a SPF of 10 would mean that you could now withstand up to 200 minutes of exposure before getting burned.

An SPF of 15 offers enough protection for most people. If you are black or very dark-skinned, you still need sunscreen if you will be out for an hour or more in intense sunlight. But if you're fair-skinned, have blue eyes, freckles, and either blond or red hair, you can get a bad burn even with an application of SPF 15 sunscreen, because you don't have the proper skin pigmentation needed to protect you.

Even the highest-rated sunscreen agent allows some solar radiation to penetrate the skin, so to be on the safe side, I've switched to a "broad spectrum" sunscreen with an SPF of 30 or more that will keep out not only the sunburn-causing UV-B rays, but the UV-A rays as well, which penetrate the deeper layers of the skin. I recommend these broad-spectrum sunscreens for their double protection.

When I choose a sunscreen, I want one that goes on easily and stays on when I perspire or go swimming. Most sunscreens in the 25–45 SPF range now meet these criteria.

Whenever I plan to go out for extended periods for sports or gardening, I always use a sunscreen. After showering in the morning, I lather down with the sunscreen right after drying off. With the skin cool and dry, the lotion penetrates readily, dries quickly, and puts a nice plasticized base on the surface of the skin.

For trouble areas such as the nose and lips, you can use sunblocks containing zinc oxide or titanium dioxide. Although these creams are messy to use and look awful, they do prevent any sunlight from reaching the skin. However, due to the sophistication levels of leading sunscreens, I don't think most people need to use these total sunblocks anymore.

Sunscreens can bring on adverse skin reactions in some people. Symptoms include itching, swelling, tingling, or a rash. The ingredient that causes the problem is PABA (para-aminobenzoic acid), a major sunscreen agent. A very small percentage of people will also be allergic to the benzophenone found in most sunscreens. As a reliable substitute, look for sunscreens marked "PABA-free" on the label.

Treatment

When I start to get pink or can feel a burn coming on, I immediately take 2 aspirin, and take 2 more every two to three hours, for a maximum of 8 aspirin. If the burn is a bad one, follow this regimen for twenty-four hours. The trick is to start taking aspirin as soon as you think you've been burned. If you wait until the next morning, it's too late.

The fact that aspirin provides some relief from pain is secondary. The primary reason to take aspirin is its ability to trigger a process that blocks a biochemical reaction that causes the skin to redden, and it helps shut down the sun's damage to the skin. Researchers aren't sure if it also prevents damage to the skin's DNA, but it

may. For children with sunburn, use pediatric dosages. If you can't take aspirin, I recommend acetaminophen or ibuprofen, but they don't work quite so well, because they're missing some of the vital blocking agents.

Don't apply any of the anesthetic sprays that are on the market. They may provide temporary relief, but they dry out the skin and can delay recovery as well. The sprays can also cause the skin to lose even more elasticity than the sunburn has caused.

For temporary relief of sunburn pain, place a cool, wet washcloth on the burned area and follow this up several times throughout the day. A lukewarm bath or shower also may be helpful to help put moisture back into the skin.

For safe relief from sunburn pain there is a natural home remedy that I find soothes the burn and promotes healing. It comes from the leaf juice of the aloe vera, a common plant found all over the Southwest. In fact, for years many people in the Southwest have used it for all kinds of skin problems from cuts to burns. Cut the fresh leaf and squeeze out the juice and apply it to the burned area like a lotion. This not only reduces the pain, but has an anti-inflammatory effect not unlike steroids.

Outside the Southwest, you can buy aloe vera plants at a nursery and keep them in your house for all kinds of skin problems, which is what I do. If you get a serious sunburn and can't find an aloe vera, then concentrated aloe vera gel sold in pharmacies is recommended.

A good warning signal that will remind you to put on sunscreen and protect yourself from the sun's potent rays is your shadow. Whenever you notice that your shadow is shorter than your body length, lather up with sunscreen. In addition, wear a broad-brimmed hat to shield your face and a long-sleeved shirt.

Cause for Concern

If you have been badly burned by the sun and have bright red, tender, painful skin and large blisters that weep and ooze, you have a serious second-degree burn, sometimes referred to as sun-poisoning, and you need to contact your dermatologist (see BURNS, page 171). After examination, the doctor may remove the fluid from the blisters and prescribe a potent oral topical steroid such as prednisone for five to seven days.

WHAT TO DO

- Apply sunscreen with SPF 15 or higher 30 minutes before going outside. Reapply as needed.
- Wear a wide-brimmed hat and long-sleeved shirt if you are especially sensitive to the sun.
- When you are sunburned, take 2 aspirin tablets every two hours, for a maximum eight hours.
- Apply aloe vera juice or gel to sunburned areas.

WARTS

Joseph P. Bark, M.D.

Dr. Bark is chairman of the Dermatology Department, St. Joseph's Hospital, Lexington, Kentucky

Warts come from the human papilloma virus, or from one of its forty-eight different subtypes, and enter the skin by direct contact. They thrive in moist environments. Once on the skin these viruses develop into nodules, usually gray-colored, benign protuberances that are highly contagious and easily spread by skin contact. Some warts will disappear over time if the immune system recognizes it as a virus and produces an antibody, but this is very rare. Warts are most effectively treated and removed by a dermatologist.

Warts are found in multiples, don't bleed or itch, and with the exception of the plantar wart on the foot, don't cause pain.

They are most commonly found on the fingers, hands, and soles of the feet. On the hands they are pale with a roughened appearance. Skin lines tend to go around them rather than through them. On the neck and face, warts tend to be small and smooth, while the painful plantar wart found on the ball or heel of the foot has the roughened look of a callus.

Children and teenagers are usually affected by warts because their still-developing immune system doesn't recognize or fight the wart virus. This changes as they age. The best precaution against plantar warts is not to go barefoot in locker rooms, poolside, or in hotels. The seemingly skimpy protection offered by wearing flip-flops or other sandals is actually all that's needed because it keeps the skin away from the wart virus.

Treatment

Home wart removal remedies sold OTC are popular, but there really is no effective self-treatment for warts. Popular OTC products containing salicylic acid, which are designed to soften and dissolve warts, are actually harmful because they delay people from seeking proper treatment and often cause skin irritation.

Cause for Concern

The real hazard comes when you *think* you have a wart and treat it with these OTC products, only to later find it isn't a wart, but a skin cancer. If you have a growth on your skin and aren't sure what it is, make an appointment with a dermatologist, have it diagnosed, confirmed, and treated.

Genital warts, also caused by the papilloma virus, are often transmitted by sexual contact. These soft, moist, pink or red warts should never be ignored because it's now believed they are influential in the development of cervical cancer. They appear singularly or in clusters. Seek treatment from your dermatologist at the first sign of any genital warts.

What the Doctor Will Do

The most common treatment a doctor will use to remove warts is cryotherapy, a quick and efficient office procedure that usually requires no anesthesia. Liquid nitrogen at minus 320 degrees is placed on the wart to freeze it. This may sting a bit and make a little red spot that will blister over the next couple of days. As the blister raises up, the virus is shed from the skin, and the wart goes away.

Other removal methods include lasers, or burning them off with electrical current. Doctors also use transdermal skin patches for the painful plantar wart found on the sole of the foot. These adhesive patches impregnated with salicyclic acid are put directly over the wart and deliver a regulated dose through the skin over the next few hours. Several applications are needed to eliminate the wart.

For small flat warts that are found on the face or other soft skin areas, tretinoin, or Retin-A, the vitamin A acid derivative, will sometimes be used in conjunction with a more powerful anticancer drug called Efudex. Once or twice daily the two creams are applied to the wart and produce an intense redness and irritation. When followed closely by a dermatologist, this treatment can result in complete resolution of the problem without any scarring.

WHAT TO DO

- Wart virus thrives in moist environments. Wear sandals or shower slippers at poolside, in locker rooms, and in hotels.
- Change your footwear regularly if you perspire heavily.
- Do not bite or cut a wart in an attempt to remove it. This spreads the wart virus.
- Do not use OTC remedies for warts. They are ineffective and may cause irritation or scarring.

- Warts are best treated by a dermatologist.
- Seek treatment immediately at the first sign of a genital wart. These warts are now linked with the onset of cervical cancer.

WRINKLES

John E. Sherman, M.D.

Dr. Sherman is assistant clinical professor of surgery, Mount Sinai School of Medicine, and a board-certified plastic surgeon in New York City

Wrinkles, the thin, creased, and sagging skin that's especially noticeable on the face, neck, and hands, are the sometimes not-so-subtle reminders of aging. Wrinkling is mainly caused by too much sun over the years, by the downward tug of gravity on the skin, genetics, and, of course, by aging.

Typically, as a person ages, the sweat and oil glands of the skin become less numerous and smaller in size. This causes the skin to lose moisture and dry out, and it soon begins to sag in places where the collagen, the elastic fibers that support the skin, has weakened the most. The skin around the eyelids, jaw, and neck is especially thin, and therefore more naturally prone to sagging.

Much of wrinkling is already predetermined by the genetic pattern passed on to you by your parents. Although you had no choice in the matter of parents and genes, there are several things you can do to delay the onset, or degree, of skin wrinkling.

Prevention

First, don't smoke. In addition to damaging the lungs, the nicotine in tobacco is a vasoconstrictor that decreases the amount of blood to the capillaries of the facial skin. If you smoke, you will ultimately develop facial wrinkles and harm the skin.

Of all outside forces, the sun's ultraviolet rays cause the most damage to the skin by breaking down the skin's collagen, its underlying elastic fibers. This ultimately causes the skin to sag and wrinkle. The sun is strongest between 10 A.M. and 3 P.M. If you plan to go outside for any length of time, apply sunblock with an SPF (sun protection factor) of at least 15 on your face and other exposed skin surfaces a half hour before heading out.

Besides the sun, the forces of heat, cold, and wind can also lead to wrinkling. So take steps to shield yourself, either with protective clothing or by using a skin moisturizer.

A great way to keep the skin from drying is to use a moisturizer on a regular basis after washing. A good lotion or cream applied to the dampened skin helps keep it from drying by trapping and holding the moisture on the skin surface.

There are many types of moisturizers available in the pharmacy. Be wary of those that claim (falsely) to be able to prevent wrinkling and counteract the effects of aging. Most of these expensive moisturizers do nothing more than moisturize the skin, just like their inexpensive counterparts. There is *no* nonprescription lotion or cream that can soften wrinkles or reverse the affects of aging skin.

To find a moisturizer that suits your needs, buy small sample containers of different types and see how your skin reacts to them.

What the Doctor Will Do

Wrinkles do not pose any health risk, but if wrinkling upsets you when you look in the mirror, consult a plastic surgeon in order to explore other wrinkle remedies. To obtain a list of plastic surgeons in your area certified by the American Board of Plastic Surgery, call 1-800-635-0635.

WHAT TO DO

- Don't smoke.
- Protect yourself from the sun. A half hour before going outside, make sure to apply sunblock with an SPF of at least 15 to all exposed skin surfaces.
- Protect yourself with clothing or skin moisturizer from extremes of heat, cold, and wind.
- Use a moisturizer on a regular basis after washing.

If wrinkling significantly upsets you when you look in the mirror, apply cosmetics to disguise the wrinkles temporarily or else consult with a board-certified plastic surgeon to discuss the available alternative measures.

General Problems

DOG BITE

Dighton C. Packard, M.D.

Dr. Packard is attending physician at Baylor University Medical Center in Dallas, Texas

More than 2 million dog bites, resulting in cuts or puncture wounds, are reported annually, half of the victims children. Millions of other bites or nips are thought to go unreported each year.

Treatment

The first thing to do after a dog has bitten you is to wash out the wound and the surrounding skin with running water. This will get rid of the dog's bacteria-laden saliva. Follow this by cleaning the wound with warm water and soap. As you are washing, decide whether you have a puncture wound, or if the bite has cut or torn the skin. A puncture is a hole in the skin that is deeper than it is long or wide. Dry the wound with a clean towel and cover it with a sterile bandage to prevent infection.

The main concern with a very deep puncture wound is potential bacterial infection. This has to be treated by a doctor. For a shallow puncture wound, such as a surface bite mark, scrupulous cleaning with soap and water followed up with personal observation over the next week is usually sufficient.

Additionally, a dog bite may cause pain, bleeding, and swelling. Take ibuprofen or aspirin for pain relief. Children should be given acetaminophen. To reduce swelling, apply an ice compress for 10 minutes and elevate the area higher than the level of the heart.

It's rare to get tetanus from a dog bite but possible. Tetanus is an infectious, life-threatening bacterium found in the soil that can enter the body whenever there is a puncture wound. If you haven't had a tetanus shot in the last ten years, contact your physician for a booster. Tetanus boosters last ten years. If you haven't had one in five years, it is advised to get one to keep your immunity level elevated.

Cause for Concern

If the skin has been cut or torn by a dog's bite, go to a hospital Emergency Department. After thoroughly cleaning the wound, the doctor will suture the cut and provide antibiotics to be taken over the next five to ten days. If there are multiple and deep cuts, surgery may be required.

Also, contact your physician if you have any doubts about your ability to self-treat or, if you have been shaken by the experience, feel in need of the assurance of a physician. If the wound becomes painful, red, swollen, and hot, or if you develop a fever, contact your physician.

Any dog bite carries the risk of rabies, a viral infection of the central nervous system transmitted through the bite of wild animals or dogs and cats infected with the rabies virus. Rabies is usually fatal and always painful, so if you have reason to suspect the animal is infected, you must be treated with special rabies vaccine. The rabies shot series is both life-saving and costly, ranging in price from $600 to $1,000. The vaccine is administered as six injections in the upper arm over a period of twenty-eight days. Unlike the earlier vaccine, the current vaccine has fewer side effects.

Most pets are immunized for rabies. However, if cases of rabies have been reported in your community, contact the dog's owner, check on its immunization record, and make sure the dog is observed for a ten-day period. Rabies symptoms include snapping and snarling at imaginary attackers, chasing its tail, foaming from the mouth, agitation, and partial paralysis.

If a stray dog bites you, report the incident to the animal control department. They will make efforts to locate the animal. Also, in some areas of the country, you may be required to report all pet attacks to the police department or local health department.

If attacked or even approached by a raccoon or other ordinarily nonaggressive animal (skunk, opossum, fox, porcupine, rabbit, squirrel), alert your local wildlife officer. If bitten, contact your physician immediately for treatment and advice.

Prevention

- Never leave a small child unattended with a dog, even a puppy. There have been many instances where teething puppies have severely bitten, even mauled, young children.
- When a dog growls or snarls, remain passive so you're not perceived as an invader.
- Slowly bring your arms up and cross them over your chest to protect yourself and remain completely still.
- Once a dog's aggression is defused, back away very slowly. If the dog charges again, stand still.
- Don't ever stare a dog directly in the eyes. A direct stare demands an aggressive response from the dog.
- Keep your eyes in the dog's general direction, let it sniff you; then hopefully it will trot off. Back away slowly and quietly, and then move on.
- If the dog is some distance away, bend over and pretend to pick up a stone or a stick. Seeing this may cause the dog to run away.

WHAT TO DO

- Wash the wound and surrounding skin with running water to flush away the dog's saliva.
- Clean the wound with warm water and soap.

- Dry the wound with a clean towel and cover with a sterile bandage to prevent infection.
- Apply an ice compress for 10 minutes to reduce swelling, and elevate the area higher than the level of the heart.
- Take aspirin or ibuprofen for pain relief.
- When the skin is cut or torn, a doctor's care is needed immediately.

FROSTBITE

Dennis C. Whitehead, M.D., F.A.C.E.P.

Dr. Whitehead is chief of Emergency Medicine, Dickinson County Memorial Hospital, Iron Mountain, Michigan

Frostbite is the temporary (superficial) or permanent (deep) skin tissue damage caused by prolonged skin-tissue temperature of 23 degrees F and below. Common warning signs include a progressive numbness and a loss of sensitivity to touch. The affected area will also tingle or feel as if it is burning. As the condition worsens, the pain begins to fade or eventually disappears.

The skin also changes color when exposed to extreme cold. It blanches, then may appear red, and finally white-purple if allowed to freeze. Most people say the affected body part feels "wooden," and it may appear to have a wooden texture.

Frostbite can affect any part of the body, but the tip of the nose, ear lobes and rim, fingertips, and toes are the most likely areas. In mild cases, full recovery can be expected with early treatment. Severe cases of frostbite can result in infection or gangrene, the death of some body tissue due to the lack of blood supply.

Frostbite is not a common problem, but can be a big problem for people who do not regularly experience severe cold weather, as well as for people who do winter camping, high-altitude climbing, hunting, and snowmobiling.

Frostnip, a superficial freezing of the outer layer of the skin—an early stage of frostbite—can also occur if you are exposed to cold weather. The skin turns white as blood circulation decreases, then stings, and becomes quite painful. Frostnip can occur during vigorous outdoor activity and you may not be aware of it until you stop exercising.

Treatment

When you first notice signs of frostbite, come out of the cold immediately and rewarm the affected area as rapidly as possible.

Do not rub the skin in an effort to get blood flowing back to the area. This causes friction and will destroy the already damaged skin and underlying tissue, as well as increase the risk of infection.

To thaw frostbitten skin, immerse the affected part in a bath kept at a constant temperature of 104–105 degrees F for upward of an hour. This will cause the blood vessels to dilate and circulation to return to the area.

Rapid rewarming is an intensely painful procedure. Take 2 ibuprofen, aspirin, or acetaminophen to dull the pain.

Do not smoke or chew tobacco. Nicotine constricts the blood vessels, reduces blood flow to chilled areas, and delays the healing process.

If you don't have access to warm water, stick the frozen body part under an armpit or between the thighs.

When the skin has thawed and rewarming is completed, cover the damaged skin with bandages and warm clothing. Contact your physician or go directly to the hospital's Emergency Department.

If there is any chance of refreezing a thawed body part, *do not* rewarm it in the first place. Freezing, rewarming, and freezing the skin again causes much more tissue damage than being frozen once.

As it rethaws, the skin turns red, swelling develops, and the area becomes quite painful. Dark blisters appear on the skin and continue to form over the ensuing week(s) as new skin develops.

What the Doctor Will Do

You should always see your doctor if you suspect frostbite.

- Doctors treat frostbite just like severe burns. After careful examination, pain medication, antibiotics, and, if needed, a tetanus booster are given.
- In the following week(s) the area is closely watched for signs of infection. The new skin that forms may be tender and permanently sensitive to the cold.

Prevention

- Before going outside in extremely cold weather (under 23 degrees F), apply skin moisturizer to the face, hands, and any other body part that may be exposed to the cold. This slows the loss of body heat.
- Dress warmly. Wear dry clothing, and stay out of the wind. Wear a face mask for extra protection.
- Wear heavy mittens instead of gloves in freezing cold weather. When the fingers are together in the mitten, their collective body heat keeps the hand warm.
- Children playing outside should be watched carefully to make sure that they don't lose or remove mittens or head-coverings.
- Be extremely careful when pumping gasoline into your car if the temperature is below freezing. Gasoline on exposed skin evaporates very quickly, lowers the temperature of the skin, and makes it more susceptible to frostbite.
- When you exercise in below-freezing temperatures, wear layers of clothing. The more layers you wear, the better insulated you are. The innermost garment must be nonabsorbent and loosely woven. Polypropylene and other newer synthetic fibers such as Capilene, Drylete, Thermax, and Dri-F.I.T., as well as the old standby, wool, are excellent because perspiration is drawn to the material and then is "wicked" (passed) on to the next layer. The second layer helps to trap warm air between you and the outermost layer(s). It should be made of wool or a synthetic material such as Synchilla or Polar Fleece. Your outer layer protects against the elements. It needs to be tightly woven. Gore-Tex, Durepel,

and Clima-F.I.T. are excellent, but nylon works fairly well in some instances. The outer shell should also have vents to let out perspiration and allow you to cool.

- When taking part in an outdoor winter activity, don't suddenly stop, cool down, then start up again. This puts you at risk for frostnip, hypothermia, or frostbite.

  To treat frostnip, get out of the cold and rewarm the skin by immersing it in water no hotter than 105 degrees F. A sure sign the skin is rewarming is pain in the frostnip area as the blood vessels begin to dilate in response to the warmth. The pain lasts only a few minutes.

- When you travel by car in the winter, keep a blanket or sleeping bag in the car at all times. If weather conditions force you to pull over to the side of the road, stay in the car and use the covers to keep warm. Your body temperature and breath will soon warm up the car. Periodically, start the car and turn on the heater. Don't leave the car; you put yourself at high risk.

Cause for Concern

Hypothermia is a drop in body temperature below 94 degrees F, and is usually caused by a combination of freezing temperatures and inadequate clothing protection. It may even occur indoors and is a particular problem with elderly people on fixed incomes, who keep their homes cool to save money. Some medications, such as Thorazine and Stelazine, interfere with temperature regulation and may contribute to hypothermia. Early warning signs include numbness, diminished shivering, cold skin, fatigue, a faint or slow pulse, loss of coordination, and slurred speech.

To treat hypothermia, get in a warm room and remove wet clothing. Wrap up in warm blankets or clothing. If none are available, have someone hug you.

The body needs to be warmed up from the center. Drink warm fluids like soup, coffee, or tea. *Do not* drink alcoholic beverages. Alcohol dilates the blood vessels and accelerates the loss of body temperature.

Take a warm, but not hot, bath. Hot water causes the blood vessels to enlarge, sending blood away from the inner organs to the surface of the body.

In extreme cases, where breathing has slowed or stopped, contact a doctor or get to an Emergency Department for treatment.

WHAT TO DO

- Come out of the cold and rewarm the body as rapidly as possible. But do not rewarm the skin if there is any chance of refreezing.
- Do not rub the skin.
- Immerse the affected part in a bath kept at a constant temperature of 104–105 degrees F for upward of an hour.
- Take 2 ibuprofen, aspirin, or acetaminophen to dull the pain.
- Stick the frozen body part under the armpit or between the thighs if you don't have access to hot water.
- Cover the damaged skin with bandages and warm clothing when rewarming is completed.
- Contact your physician or go to the Emergency Department for an examination and further treatment.

Frostnip, a superficial freezing of the outer layer of skin and an early stage of frostbite, will occur if you are inadequately protected and exposed to cold weather. To treat frostnip:

- Get out of the cold and rewarm the skin by immersing it in water no hotter than 105 degrees F.

HANGNAIL

Paul Kechijian, M.D.

Dr. Kechijian is associate clinical professor of Dermatology, New York University Medical Center in New York City

A hangnail may appear brittle, tough, and as hard as a fingernail, but it isn't a nail at all. It is a piece of dehydrated skin that is cracked or detached from either the cuticle or skin folds that border the fingernail. When it sticks out and gets snagged on things, it tugs and rips away from the skin.

The most common cause of a hangnail is dehydration. This typically occurs when you have your hands repeatedly in and out of water, as I do during the course of my work day. In between seeing patients, I wash my hands, which causes the skin to absorb water and swell. But as the water evaporates, the skin dries out and shrinks. Repeated swelling and shrinking eventually leads to cracking. This commonly develops at the junction where the cuticle and lateral nail fold meet each other at the rear corners of the nail.

Hangnails are a common problem not only for doctors and nurses, but for dishwashers, chefs, homemakers, or barbers—people who have their hands in and out of water all day.

Hangnails are more common in the winter months than the summer, because frigid air holds less moisture, making the air drier. Heating of homes, offices, and stores dries the air further and also draws moisture from the skin, making the skin and nails not only more prone to dryness (see DRY SKIN, page 184) but more susceptible to hangnails.

Treatment

Hangnails become a problem when people pull off dried skin—by biting it, for example. Not only is this unsanitary, but it creates the possibility of infection by transmitting germs from the mouth. Also, when you tear the skin with your teeth, you often pull it too far and end up with a larger cut that hurts and may become infected.

If you develop a cut from hangnail, take a clean piece of cotton or tissue and press it on the area until the bleeding stops. To prevent infection, put a dab of antiseptic ointment such as Polysporin on the cut and cover the area with an adhesive bandage. Whenever your hands get wet, change the bandage and reapply the antiseptic. After two or three days, the skin should be healed and the risk of infection passed. Trim away any remaining hangnail with scissors.

Cause for Concern

If the finger becomes red, swollen, and hot to the touch, contact your physician immediately. You most likely have developed an infection and need oral antibiotic treatment.

The best way to deal with a hangnail is to trim it with a pair of small, clean, sharp scissors at the outset. Cut away the dried skin right to the base.

Prevention

- To reduce hangnails in the winter, wear gloves when you're outdoors to keep your hands warm and prevent moisture from escaping.
- Every time you wash your hands, apply moisturizer. The cream will trap moisture in the skin, making it less likely to crack and form a hangnail. Petroleum jelly is excellent, but greasy. If you use it, apply it at night and wear a pair of light cotton gloves so you don't stain your bedding or night clothing.
- One inexpensive moisturizer is pure vegetable shortening. Rub it in several times daily after washing, and your hands will be well moisturized.

WHAT TO DO

- Wear gloves outdoors in the cold, winter months.
- Moisturize the hands and fingers regularly, particularly after washing them.
- If a hangnail tears and a cut develops that begins to bleed, stop the bleeding with a cotton ball, apply antiseptic ointment, and cover with an adhesive bandage. If the finger becomes swollen, red, or hot to the touch, contact your physician.

HEADACHE

Seymour Diamond, M.D.

Dr. Diamond is director, Diamond Headache Clinic; adjunct professor of pharmacology and molecular biology, Chicago Medical School; clinical associate in medicine, University of Chicago; and executive director of the National Headache Foundation

Headaches rank just after the common cold as the ailment that most bothers Americans, and for 50 million of them the headaches are so severe they consult a doctor.

Headaches are more common among women, but perhaps because men often deny they have pain. People who smoke or drink excessively are also more prone to headache distress.

Headaches can also be triggered by missing a meal, sun glare, certain odors, bad posture, medicines, or an incorrect eyeglass prescription.

Headaches are divided into two distinct categories—tension headaches and vascular headaches, which include migraine and cluster headaches. Each has a broad spectrum of causes, symptoms, and treatment.

Tension Headache

A tension headache begins when the scalp muscles tense and go into spasm. As circulation to these muscles is reduced, pain develops at the back of the head and neck, the scalp and forehead.

Prevention

- Bad posture can trigger tension headaches, a common complaint for the millions of people who use video display terminals (VDTs).
- To prevent or reduce headaches when using a VDT, equip your screen with an antiglare filter, and keep the terminal away from light coming in from windows or from overhead fluorescent lighting.
- When seated, your feet should rest comfortably on the floor, with your thighs horizontal or sloping downward at a slight angle. Keep your elbows at your sides and your wrists held out straight when you type. Shoulders should be back, and your head straight upright as you look directly at the screen. Keep material you are typing at eye level so you don't have to bend your neck as you work.
- Every hour, get up and take a break. Stretch your shoulders, neck, and lower back with gentle bending and twisting motions.

Excessive sunlight is a common tension headache trigger. Wear sunglasses if you develop headaches after being in the sun for any length of time.

Treatment

If you get tension headaches from stress, and if the headache occurs once a month or more, take one of the OTC remedies such as aspirin, acetaminophen, or ibuprofen. These medications work very well to end the pain in just a short while. Experimentation is needed here to find which drug works best for you. To avoid stomach distress, take the medicine according to directions and after eating some food.

If you don't want to use medication, there are several other effective measures you can try.

Apply cold to your head. Fill a plastic bag with ice and place it on the spot that is sore. Leave it there for 10 to 15 minutes.

Take a hot bath or a shower to relieve muscle soreness in the neck.

Gently massage your forehead and neck with the tips of your fingers.

Stretch your neck and shoulders. While sitting down, let your head drop down, with your chin resting on your chest. Then, slowly move your head in a circular motion and make several revolutions past your chest.

Exercise for headache relief is a two-edged sword. Performing some form of aerobic activity such as walking, running, or bicycling may relieve tension symptoms for 70 percent of people, but for the remaining 30 percent it could actually worsen a headache.

Regular exercise helps with stress release and keeps headaches from developing, most likely because of the release of endorphins, the body's own natural opiates, which have a sedating effect. However, if you exercise and find that a headache begins, or that it makes a previous headache feel worse, then stop exercising.

Cause for Concern

Headaches are not always benign and are often a sign of underlying problems that need to be treated by a physician. These can include high blood pressure, allergies, the flu, a middle ear infection, encephalitis, or a brain tumor.

Contact your physician if you are having daily headaches, if you take OTC medication for headache on a daily basis, if you miss work regularly because of headache, if exercise or sexual intercourse triggers headache, or if you have a severe headache accompanied by a fever and a stiff neck, which is a sign of meningitis, an inflammation of the brain lining.

For a regional referral list of neurologists, internists, and family physicians who specialize in headache treatment, contact the National Headache Foundation by calling 1-800-843-2252. In Illinois, call 1-800-523-8858.

What the Doctor Will Do

- The doctor will take a thorough medical history, perform a neurological exam to test various reflexes as well as motor, sensory, and cranial nerve function.
- Once organic disease has been ruled out, the doctor may recommend prescription medications, relaxation techniques, meditation, yoga, or self-hypnotic exercises to counteract your headaches.

- Biofeedback may also be recommended. A trained therapist connects sensors to your hand and fingers and asks you to do different relaxation techniques. The biofeedback machine then detects subtle body changes that indicate which work best for you. After a few sessions, you will no longer need the biofeedback machine to achieve relaxation.
- The doctor may gradually wean you off aspirin, ibuprofen, or acetaminophen. When these pain relievers are used continuously and then stopped, headache can easily be provoked. A gradual diminution is needed.

Migraine Headache

Migraine headache pain can range from mild to severe, last for an hour to a day or two. Migraine symptoms include nausea or vomiting, dizziness, throbbing pain that begins over one eye that soon spreads to other parts of the head, oversensitivity to light or sound, and a desire to hibernate to sleep off the pain.

Migraine headaches can begin at puberty, but most first develop in the twenties or thirties. More than three-fourths of people with migraines are women, and there is a strong genetic link. My mother-in-law had migraine headaches and now my three daughters all get them. Many female migraine sufferers will get attacks before, during, and after their menstrual periods or when they take oral contraceptives. In 70 percent of the cases, women will stop having migraines after menopause.

Other factors that lead to migraines include head injuries, stress, alcohol, and certain foods or beverages containing the protein tyramine, or food additives such as monosodium glutamate (MSG) and nitrites.

Treatment

If you have migraine headache symptoms, do not try to treat yourself. Contact a physician who specializes in treating headaches and develop a headache treatment program tailored to your needs.

Once you've been properly diagnosed by your physician, in addition to taking aspirin, acetaminophen, or ibuprofen or prescription medication for migraine pain, there are several other things you can do.

- Splash your face with cold water.
- Apply an icepack to your head.
- Drink 1–2 cups of caffeinated coffee to constrict the blood vessels.
- Lie down in a dark, quiet room and try to relax through meditation, using biofeedback techniques, or sleep.

What the Doctor Will Do

After ruling out any underlying organic causes, the doctor may prescribe antidepressant drugs or muscle relaxants, or medication to constrict the blood vessels and hopefully prevent migraines from developing.

- If you have frequent migraines, the doctor may prescribe propanolol (Inderal) to be taken daily as a prophylactic.
- Recommend relaxation training such as meditation, yoga, or biofeedback.
- Recommend you go on a tyramine-free diet. Tyramine is a chemical found in many common foods, but is not handled properly by most people prone to migraines.

Foods rich in tyramine include cheeses such as Boursault, Camembert, cheddar, Stilton, blue, Gruyère, mozzarella, Parmesan, Romano, Roquefort, and ricotta.

- Recommend you keep a daily food diary and note your reactions to different foods to determine which foods trigger migraines.
- Caffeine is a vasoconstrictor, which, if consumed in excessive quantities, may cause a rebound headache. Caffeine-containing beverages (coffee, tea, colas) and medications should be limited.
- For severe attacks, the physician may prescribe a compound containing ergot, a drug that works well in migraine treatment. For those patients who are not able to use ergots, a drug containing isometheptene (Midrin) may be used.

Cluster Headache

Cluster headaches are the most painful of all headaches. Some people bang their heads against a wall to relieve pain, others talk of shooting themselves, while a small group of despondent people actually do take their lives to get relief from the agony.

Cluster headaches strike 90 percent more males than females. This excruciating, one-sided headache centers around one eye or its surrounding area. When it strikes, it causes a constriction of the pupil, tearing of the eye, flushing of the face, and nasal congestion. Cluster headaches get their name because they come without warning in a cluster and occur at the same time of day or night. They continue like clockwork day after day for weeks or months. The pain lasts from thirty to forty-five minutes, and usually no longer than two hours. Cluster headaches can go away on their own, only to return months or years later with the same intensity.

There is no clear cause for cluster headaches, but smoking and excessive drinking seem to stimulate them. Aspirin and acetaminophen have no effect on cluster headaches.

What the Doctor Will Do

A doctor's counsel is essential.

- The doctor may prescribe prednisone, a corticosteroid medication, to break the cluster cycle. Methysergide or lithium are also used in treatment.
- One of the most effective treatments is to inhale 100 percent oxygen over a 15-minute period.

WHAT TO DO

- Make sure your work station is properly adjusted and your sitting position is comfortable.
- Wear sunglasses on bright, sunny days.
- Take an OTC medication such as acetaminophen, aspirin, or ibuprofen, but not on a daily basis.

- Apply either a cold or hot compress to the painful area.
- Massage and gently stretch your neck and shoulders.
- Exercise regularly.

A migraine headache typically occurs on one side of the head, affects women primarily. In classical migraine, its onset is often signaled 15 to 30 minutes before by an aura, bright spots, or jagged lines that appear in the line of vision. Patients with common migraine may have a premonition of an impending attack. Don't treat yourself for a migraine headache. After being properly diagnosed by a physician, the following steps may help reduce the frequency or severity of migraine headache:

- Go on a tyramine-free diet and maintain a regular meal schedule.
- Take OTC or prescription medications but not on a daily basis.
- Apply an ice pack to your head.
- Lie down in a dark room and try to relax.

Cluster headache is the most painful and debilitating of all headaches. For counseling and relief, contact a physician who specializes in headaches.

INSOMNIA

Cheryl M. Carlucci, M.D.

Dr. Carlucci is clinical assistant professor of Neurology at the Albany Medical Center, and medical director of the Capital Region Sleep–Wake Disorder Center in Albany, New York

Temporary difficulty in falling asleep, or the inability to stay asleep once you are in bed, is the most common sleep complaint in this country. At least 40 percent of the American population has problems with insomnia at some time during the year, while 15 percent suffer from it on a chronic basis.

Symptoms manifested during waking hours can include any or all of the following: fatigue, difficulty in concentration, lack of coordination, numbness, irritability, weariness, slurred speech, headaches, and blurred vision.

Insomnia is not a disease in and of itself, but a symptom of a temporary or long-term problem such as too much anxiety or stress (see STRESS, page 238), depression, excitement, the hormonal changes of menopause, jet lag (see JET LAG, page 227), grief, reaction to a medication or food product, or from the overuse of caffeine or alcohol products. No illness is specifically linked with not getting enough sleep, but some research suggests insomnia can diminish the body's immune system.

Most of us need about eight hours of sleep a night, but many people try to get away with less. A tip-off that you are sleep deprived is when you fall asleep as soon as you go to bed.

Many times insomnia develops when children or adults have difficulty surrendering to sleep out of fear that their safety is somehow in jeopardy during sleep. They are afraid to go to sleep. Counseling can cure insomnia and natural sleep can return.

Treatment

Whenever you experience problems with insomnia, don't stay in bed tossing and turning. Instead, get up and take your mind off trying to fall asleep by reading a book or newspaper. When you finally begin to feel drowsy, go back to bed.

I occasionally have insomnia. However, before I get out of bed, I ask myself, "Could I really get up right now?" If the answer is no, it means I'm probably in a twilight state between sleep and wakefulness. Realizing I'm not ready to get up allows me to let go of the wakefulness, and in a matter of minutes I'm sound asleep again.

Make sure your bed is not contributing to your insomnia. If you wake up with a backache or don't feel refreshed after sleeping, you will come to associate your bed with a torture chamber. Switch to a mattress or bed that is more comfortable.

The sleeping environment has to promote relaxation. If the room is too hot or too dry, your nasal passages can become dry and can interfere with sleep. Check the ventilation and humidity level in your bedroom. Also, make the room as dark and as quiet as possible.

Sleep is never as restorative as it should be if you hear a lot of noise in your bedroom. The worst type is intermittent noise from an airplane, a fire engine, or loud truck. You may not actually be aware of waking, but these noises will cause arousals that fragment your sleep. The more fragmentation, the sleepier you will feel the next day.

If you're constantly bothered by noise, wear ear plugs. I prefer the soft, silicone plugs to the foam or wax types because they work better at blocking sound. These small, inexpensive devices are sold in most pharmacies.

Many people have difficulty sleeping because they wait until nighttime to focus on problems or crises that occurred during the day. The end result is that suppressed problems "come out at night."

Worrying harms your sleep. Set aside a time period of at least 30 minutes to an hour each night before you go to bed and try to work out your problems. Keep a journal and sketch out your trouble spots. Next, write out how you plan to attack your problem and come up with workable solutions. When it's finally time for bed, you can sleep easier because you know that you've made positive efforts to take care of these issues. In a sense, you've "laid them to rest."

Exercise on a regular basis may promote better sleep by helping you to relax. Several hours before bedtime, go for a walk or a run, or participate in your favorite sport or fitness activity. There are no hard and fast rules about when to exercise. In general, exercising right before bedtime is invigorating and may keep you awake. Find out what works best for you.

An occasional nap may refresh you during daylight hours, but when it lasts more than 30 minutes, it may contribute to insomnia.

A warm bath just before bedtime can work wonders because as you relax in the tub, the hot water warms up your blood and brain, which can also make you feel sleepy.

Avoid eating a large meal just before bedtime. Although it may make you drowsy at first, all that energy in the food will enter your system two to three hours later, and you may wake up in the middle of the night or end up having a restless night's sleep.

Instead of a large meal, eat a carbohydrate-rich food snack like a bowl of natural-grain (and low sugar) cereal just before bedtime. The carbohydrates may make you drowsy, and the slow metabolism of the complex carbohydrates will prevent a major drop in blood glucose levels during the night.

Sex is a great energy burner, and for many people sexual activity carried on at bedtime offers not only a great sense of physical release but acts as a natural sleeping pill as well.

Sleep researchers used to say that the bed was strictly for sleeping and that you shouldn't read or watch TV in bed. However, some people find reading even a few pages of a book or magazine helps them go to sleep. It makes me go to sleep quicker than anything else.

Caffeine will stay in the system for as long as fourteen hours after you eat or drink a caffeinated product. In many cases the drug, which is found in colas, coffee, tea, and chocolate, has its greatest effect in the middle of the night when the body is sleeping.

If you find that caffeine disturbs your sleep, don't take any after noon. If you are still bothered by insomnia, eliminate it gradually by reducing your intake over a period of four to five days. Caffeine can be an addictive drug, so never go cold turkey; this may lead to headaches. Start by eliminating the last cup in the evening, then stop after your midafternoon coffee break. Next, cut out your lunchtime coffee, and finally don't drink coffee at breakfast. Once you've eliminated coffee, you should sleep more soundly.

Avoid all alcohol before bedtime if you find it disturbs your sleep. Alcohol is a short-acting depressant that makes you feel tired and brings on an unnaturally induced sleep. You'll sleep for a few hours but then may wake up suddenly because the depressant effect of the alcohol has worn off. Also, alcohol can be dangerous for people with sleep apnea (see SNORING, page 236).

Stop smoking. Nicotine found in cigarettes can be a powerful stimulant and may disturb the quality of your sleep. Smoking also irritates the tissue in the upper airway. This can make snoring and sleep apnea worse.

Counting sheep as you lie in bed is not recommended. Counting requires you to focus the brain on a specific activity, and sleep is a defocusing of mental activity. When I'm troubled by mild insomnia, I think of myself in a pleasant spot such as the beach. I don't focus on any details, but try to experience the warmth of the sun and the relaxation I feel as I lie on the sand listening to the waves.

Avoid sleeping pills whenever possible. However, for infrequent cases of insomnia there is a role for these drugs. If you travel and can't sleep in a new environment, or if you're under acute stress, then sleeping pills can be helpful. By reducing mental activity, these medications allow sleep to occur when it otherwise would not. Don't use them for more than two nights, or you may develop chronic insomnia.

Cause for Concern

Both prescription and nonprescription sleeping pills can lead to depression if taken over an extended period of time—a month or so. As tolerance develops, you will require more of the drug to produce the same effect. Benzodiazepine, the drug in many prescription sleeping pills, can stay in your system for quite some time. They can make you feel groggy and fatigued during the day. Once you stop taking the medication after prolonged use, you will find you cannot sleep without the medication, even though it no longer helps you fall asleep quickly. If this happens, you've become addicted to the medication.

What the Doctor Will Do

If these sleep techniques fail to curb your insomnia, see your physician for a check-up to rule out any underlying medical problems. A referral to a sleep specialist or sleep center may be necessary. In some cases of insomnia, sleep studies may be done to determine the cause of the insomnia.

The American Sleep Disorders Association, 604 Second Street, S.W., Rochester, MN 55902, (507) 287-6006, can provide nationwide referrals to sleep specialists (doctors trained in neurology, psychology, or pulmonary medicine) and put you in touch with sleep centers in your area.

WHAT TO DO

- Keep regular bedtimes.
- Don't allow yourself extra hours of sleep on the weekend.
- Don't stay in bed tossing and turning. Get out of bed and do something to take your mind off trying to fall asleep.
- Make the room as dark and as quiet as possible.
- Don't bring your problems to bed. Set aside a period each night before bedtime to work them out.
- Exercise during the day can help sleeplessness. At least four hours before bedtime, participate in your favorite sport, exercise, or fitness activity.
- Avoid naps during the day.
- Don't eat a large meal before bedtime.
- Eat a carbohydrate-rich food for a snack if you're hungry before bedtime.
- Don't take any caffeinated product after

noon, or eliminate it gradually from your diet if caffeine causes insomnia for you.

- Stop smoking.
- Don't count sheep. Use mental imagery to transport yourself to a pleasant, peaceful place and ease yourself into sleep.

- Avoid sleeping pills.
- If these sleep remedies fail to curb your insomnia and it interferes with your work or enjoyment, contact a sleep specialist or a certified sleep center for assistance.

JET LAG

Daniel R. Wagner, M.D.

Dr. Wagner is a chronobiologist and assistant professor of clinical neurology, psychiatry, neurology, and neuroscience at the New York Hospital–Cornell Medical Center in White Plains, New York

Jet lag, a common problem for long-distance air travelers, can wipe out even the best-laid business or social plans. This physically and mentally debilitating condition often occurs after the victim has traveled rapidly across three or more time zones and then tries to acclimate sleeping, eating, and waking habits to the new locale.

The standard rule of thumb is that for each time zone crossed, one day is needed for the body to adapt to the change in daily routines.

Traveling to the east and forcing your internal body clock to reset forward shortens your day, while heading west is less of a problem because it lengthens your day in the direction of its natural internal cycle. Flying north to south has no effect.

High-speed, long-distance travel forces a change in the timing of your normal sleeping-waking-eating schedule. This clashes with dozens of internal bodily functions that occur each day during a circadian schedule.

Circadian rhythms are the daily body cycles, the internal clock that regulates most of our physiological functions. Fiddle with these natural rhythms by staying up later than usual, and you can disrupt normal heart rate and body temperature, as well as hormonal and nervous system activities. Many times, it can take seven or more days for these bodily rhythms to adjust to their normal daily timing.

Jet lag symptoms can also include deep fatigue, daytime sleepiness, waking up too early, and an inability to get back to sleep. You may begin to feel irritable, tense, and out of sorts. These symptoms can range from mild to severe depending on your age, distance traveled, and how well you prepared for your trip. Mental alertness, athletic ability, and strength are also affected.

In rare cases, extreme mood disorders may develop. Depression can be triggered when traveling from east to west, while a manic state can be caused in some people when traveling west to east.

Prevention

Jet lag cannot be entirely prevented, but you can reduce its severity.

Analyze your purpose in making the journey, and give yourself time to adapt to the new time zone after you arrive.

When I travel across country from New York to California, I sleep on Central time, which is an hour later than my home time, Eastern. By sleeping on Central time throughout the trip, I have only a one-hour time adjustment to make upon returning home.

If I have to be in California only a short while, but need to be especially alert when I return home, then I won't time-shift at all. I'll stay on East Coast time the entire period that I'm in California.

For a time shift of ten to fourteen hours required for a trip to Japan or Australia, it takes up to two weeks to resynchronize your internal clock to local time, but acclimation can be speeded up by switching your sleep patterns.

The human sleep-wake cycle has two "sleepy" phases, and by not napping during the daytime upon arrival in the Orient, you should be able to move your main sleep period into the afternoon "sleepy zone."

A trip to Europe is the toughest for me because it involves time shifts of five to nine hours. Several days before leaving, I change eating and sleeping schedules by going to bed an hour earlier each night and arising an hour earlier in the morning. For the return leg of the trip, several days before departure, I go to bed an hour later and arise an hour later each day. This helps shift the internal clock back toward New York time.

Diet may help reduce jet lag. However, tests of the popular "antijet-lag diet" have not conclusively shown that a person's circadian rhythms will adapt more readily to a new time zone by a change in eating habits.

The quicker you can adapt your eating, work, exercise, and sleeping habits to the local schedule, the quicker jet lag symptoms will disappear. Therefore, don't nap in your hotel room immediately upon arrival. Go outside into the sunlight, even if you feel like a zombie. Light hitting the eye is one of the main mechanisms for resetting the internal clock.

Physical activity also helps synchronize your internal clock. As soon as possible after your arrival, go for a walk or take part in your favorite exercise. The object is not to maintain your regular workout regime from home, but simply to move around. A fast two-mile jog in a London park when your body thinks you should be sleeping in New York is usually a no-win situation. Therefore, cut your pace and distance, or slow down and walk instead.

Age is also a factor in whether or not you will develop jet lag symptoms. Most time shifts are not all that deleterious before the age of thirty. However, our lab studies show that people over age thirty have reduced sleep efficiency as long as ten days after a single six-hour time shift.

Therefore, if you are in this age category and need to travel, prepare for jet lag and don't ignore it once it hits. Ignoring jet lag will only create additional problems, and bring on other problems associated with sleep deprivation.

WHAT TO DO

- Prepare properly for your trip. Set aside the first day to get used to your change in daily routine.
- For a business trip from one coast to the other, follow a sleep schedule *as if* you were in the Central or Mountain time zone in order to avoid jet lag on either end of the trip.
- After arriving in Japan or Australia from the United States, don't nap during the days after arrival. Go to bed and get up at the sleep-wake schedule of the new time zone. Spend as much of the first two or three days outside in the light.
- For European jaunts, start going to bed an hour earlier and arising an hour earlier each day several days prior to departure.
- Resist the urge to nap following a daytime arrival. Go outside in the sunshine.
- Go for a walk or take part in your favorite exercise or sports activity soon after arrival, and on subsequent mornings as well.

LYME DISEASE

Raymond J. Dattwyler, M.D.

Dr. Dattwyler is associate professor of medicine at the State University of New York at Stony Brook, and director of the Lyme Disease Clinic

Lyme disease, named after the town of Lyme, Connecticut, where many cases were first diagnosed in 1975, is a bacterial infection transmitted to humans by a tick bite. These minuscule deer ticks are responsible for spreading the disease in forty-six states, infecting well over 8,000 people in 1990. Connecticut, New Jersey, Wisconsin, Rhode Island, and California have most of the reported cases; New York leads with over 4,000 cases annually.

The ticks live in grasses and low vegetation found in wooded areas and near the beach. When a human or pet such as a dog or cat pass by, these parasites simply attach themselves and begin to live off the blood of their new warm-blooded host. In some areas, upward of 50 percent of the ticks carry the Lyme disease bacteria, but in most places, the percentage of infected ticks is much lower.

Lyme disease received a lot of media hype in the 1980s that often bordered on hysteria. When Lyme disease went untreated—as it often did in early days because many doctors couldn't properly diagnose or treat it—it often progressed to chronic arthritis, and sometimes to meningitis and Bell's palsy, which is a partial paralysis of the face.

Today we have effective treatment for Lyme disease. If detected early, nearly 100 percent of Lyme disease cases are successfully combated over a two- to three-week period with simple oral antibiotics such as tetracycline. However, if the disease is allowed to progress before treatment is begun, the cure rate dips to approximately

90 percent, and the residual problems of hot or swollen joints and chronic arthritis may linger, depending on how long you had the disease.

Symptoms develop anywhere from three days to a month after being bitten by a tick. They include viruslike symptoms of headache, sore throat, fever, joint and muscle aches, and fatigue that lasts for about a week. In half to three-quarters of the cases a unique telltale red rash develops around the bite site. Usually, the rash is large, 3 or more inches in diameter. It has a raised edge and a pale center that becomes larger over a period of days and then begins to fade.

If you are positive that you've been bitten by a tick, and have a rash or other symptoms, contact your physician.

Lyme disease can be difficult to diagnose because symptoms vary from person to person, and can easily fit the description of other common ailments. To make matters worse, the blood test currently used for Lyme disease is so inaccurate that approximately 2–8 percent of healthy people test positive for it. Newer, more reliable blood tests will be available soon that will make definitive testing possible.

In the meantime, if you suspect Lyme disease, a cautious and careful evaluation should be made by a rheumatologist or an infectious disease expert in order to make a proper diagnosis.

Prevention

- June, July, and August are prime tick months. If you go for a walk in known tick areas, stay in the middle of the walking trails.
- Weather permitting, cover up your body as much as possible when you go out. Tuck your pants into your socks.
- It's easier to spot a tick on light-colored material, so wear light-colored pants and a tightly woven, long-sleeved shirt with the collar and sleeves buttoned.
- Spray any standard insect repellent containing 30 percent deet (N, N–M–diethyltoluamide) on exposed skin or 0.5 percent permethrin on clothing.
- Dogs and cats pick up ticks too and should be checked carefully before they are let into the house. For added protection, use a tick or flea collar. Animals can get Lyme disease, but as far as it is known, cannot transmit it to humans directly.
- If you fear you may have been exposed, inspect yourself from head to toe when you get home. Have someone check the back of your head and neck.

The deer tick is flat and small as a poppy seed, has eight legs, and may look like a tiny mole or blood blister on your skin. Since ticks are parasites, they will go anywhere on your body in search of a meal, so be sure to check carefully, even in the groin area and under your arms.

- If you find a tick on your skin, remove it with fine-point tweezers as close to the skin as possible. Grasping the tick by the head, pull it straight out.
- Save the tick in alcohol and date the container for a doctor to identify later if you develop Lyme symptoms.
- Wash off the bite area with soap and water and then apply an antiseptic such as rubbing alcohol.
- It takes at least twenty-four hours for a tick feeding on you to transmit Lyme infection. If the tick is engorged with blood when you discover it, assume it's been there for many hours, and your

likelihood of contracting Lyme disease is high.
- If the tick is still flat, it may not have had a chance to dig into you. In either case, remove the tick properly, and show it to your physician if you later develop Lyme symptoms.

WHAT TO DO

- Stay in the middle of walking trails in the woods when you go for walks in known tick areas.
- Cover up your body as much as possible whenever you go out in the woods.

- Tuck your pants into your socks.
- Wear a light-colored, tightly woven, long-sleeved shirt with the collar and sleeves buttoned.
- Spray insect repellent containing 30 percent deet on exposed skin or use a spray containing 0.5 percent permethrin on clothing.
- Give yourself a head to toe inspection for ticks when you get home. Picking the ticks off prevents Lyme disease.
- If you are positive that you've been bitten by a tick, and you develop typical Lyme disease symptoms, contact a rheumatologist or infectious disease expert.

NOSEBLEED

Michael O. Fleming, M.D.

Dr. Fleming is a physician in private family practice in Shreveport, Louisiana

Everyone experiences a nosebleed from time to time. The cause may be an impact to the nose, but many times the nose bleeds because of nasal congestion due to a nasal allergy, strep throat, a sinus infection, or a cold that irritates and weakens the delicate nasal lining. In some adults, especially those taking aspirin or anticoagulants, the bleeding may start spontaneously. However, the main cause of nosebleeds is people picking or irritating the small blood vessels just inside the nose. If you pick, rub, or irritate these veins, they can break open and bleed.

Treatment

To stop a common nosebleed, apply pressure to the dividing wall between the nostrils. First, sit or stand upright with the head slightly tilted forward to lower blood pressure to the head, and prevent the escaping blood from flowing down the throat.

Take your thumb and forefinger and forcefully grab the front of your nose. Press hard enough so that the nostrils are pressed tightly against the septum. You know you have applied enough pressure if you look in a mirror and see the skin blanch. Breathe through your mouth and continue to apply this pressure for one minute by the clock.

Most of the time, this pressure is sufficient to cause the blood to clot and stop the nosebleed. If the nose continues to bleed, apply pressure for another minute. If the bleeding still continues unabated after 15 minutes of steady pressure, contact your physician.

Once the bleeding has stopped, don't blow your nose for several hours or you may cause it to bleed again. Apply an antibiotic ointment to a cotton-tipped applicator and gently rub it on the inside of your nose. The antibiotic will help destroy any germs, while the ointment will help keep the nasal lining moist. Reapply the ointment several times a day for several days, especially before going to bed at night. Many people tend to rub their noses unconsciously in their sleep, especially children. If the nasal lining is dry and unprotected, it can easily begin to bleed again.

Nosebleeds tend to recur because, although the tissue quickly heals, it takes more than a week for the area to heal completely. In the meantime, if you rub the nose hard, sneeze, blow your nose, or stick your finger in your nose to scratch or remove dried crusts of mucus inside the nose, you effectively remove the healing tissue and the bleeding can start all over again.

Prevention

Air in pressurized airplane cabins can cause nosebleeds, especially on transcontinental or intercontinental flights. The dry air irritates the nasal lining.

- Before takeoff, apply a small coating of petroleum jelly with a cotton-tipped applicator to the inside of your nostrils. Reapply it as needed during the flight.

- Stay well hydrated by drinking plenty of nonalcoholic, noncaffeinated fluids in flight.

Winter is a common time for nosebleeds because of the low humidity, frigid temperatures, and the prevalence of colds, flu, and other viruses that can cause nasal irritation. Since homes are kept warm in the winter—many times too warm and dry for the sake of your nose and skin—keep your bedroom well humidified, keep your window open, and if necessary, use a humidifier or vaporizer.

Cause for Concern

Nosebleeds can develop in the rear part of the nose. Blood will typically flow backward and down the throat instead of out the nose. Applying pressure to the nostrils will not stop the flow of blood, and blood loss could be substantial. You must see your doctor or head to the Emergency Department in order to be treated.

In middle-aged people, this type of spontaneous bleeding is often related to high blood pressure that is not well controlled, or not yet diagnosed. A nosebleed stemming from the back of the nose can also result from hemophilia, which is a bleeding disorder, leukemia, and other bleeding disorders related to low platelet levels or blood clotting.

If you can't stop your nose from bleeding, if it starts bleeding after a head injury but no accompanying injury to the nose, or if you have frequent nosebleeds and you suspect that it's due to something other than a nasal irritation, contact your physician or go to the hospital Emergency Department.

What the Doctor Will Do

- The doctor will pack the nose with gauze at the point where the back of the nose meets the back of the throat. This will put pressure on the damaged artery and stop the bleeding.
- For persistent bleeding, the nostril may first be anesthetized and a catheter then inserted. As the catheter fills with blood, pressure is applied to the artery and bleeding stops.
- In the case of head injury, X rays will be taken to see if there is a possible skull fracture.

WHAT TO DO

- Sit or stand upright with the head slightly tilted forward.

- Forcefully grab the front of your nose and with the thumb and forefinger, press hard enough so the nostrils are compressed tightly against the septum.
- Breathe through your mouth and continue to apply pressure for one minute.
- Don't blow your nose for several hours or do any strenuous activity once the bleeding has stopped.
- Apply an antibiotic ointment to the inside of your nose.
- Keep your bedroom well humidified.
- If you can't stop your nose from bleeding, if it starts bleeding after a head injury, or if you suspect the bleeding is due to something other than an irritation or minor blow, contact your physician or go to the hospital Emergency Department.

SNAKE BITE

Earl Schwartz, M.D.

Dr. Schwartz is chairman of the Department of Emergency Medicine of the Bowman Gray School of Medicine of Wake Forest University in Winston-Salem, North Carolina

Each year in this country approximately 37,000 people are bitten by nonpoisonous snakes, while 8,000 others are bitten by poisonous ones. When proper action is taken, recovery from a poisonous snake bite is complete. Death from a poisonous snake bite is extremely rare.

There are two distinct classes of poisonous snakes in the United States. The first is pit vipers, with their triangular heads, elongated fangs, elliptical pupils, and a heat-sensing pit—an indentation at the front of the face. The rattlesnake, copperhead, and cottonmouth—known as the water moccasin in some areas—are all pit vipers.

When a pit viper strikes, it injects venom through the skin with its long hypodermiclike fangs. The venom attacks the circulatory system, causing you to bleed and your blood pressure to drop. There is a great deal of pain soon after. Some liken the pain to a hot iron on the skin. This is followed by numbness and swelling. In moderate snake bites, there may be some nausea and vomiting, while severe poisoning brings on a total body swelling that will turn the skin blue. Blistering and severe pain are other common symptoms.

The severity of symptoms depends on how much venom was injected, and if it is injected into the bloodstream. With a major bite, symptoms develop in minutes, while a minor bite can take an hour or more before you notice any sign of trouble.

Pit vipers do not always inject venom when they bite. A snake can control the amount of venom it releases, which is usually enough to immobilize or kill its prey, so that it can be eaten. The snake has no intention of eating a human, so if it injects any poison when it attacks, it is often just enough to scare you away.

The coral snake, found in the western and southeastern parts of the country, is alone in the other class of poisonous snakes found in this country. This first cousin to the cobra is slender and about a yard long, and it has red, yellow, and black bands circling its body, making it look similar to several nonvenomous snakes. One way to differentiate the coral snake from the others is by this ditty: "Red on yellow will kill a fellow." The bright red and yellow bands of the coral snake abut each other. But anyone inexpert in snake lore is wise to avoid *all* snakes banded in red, yellow, and black.

The coral snake has a small mouth, so when it strikes, it's likely to hold on and chew a toe or finger. The poison runs down a groove in its tooth—it has very short fangs—and enters the superficial wound it has created. The venom affects the nervous system and causes paralysis within hours if left untreated. This paralysis can be fatal if it reaches the respiratory system.

If you are bitten by any poisonous snake, go to the nearest hospital Emergency Department as quickly as possible. However, before you go, there are several things you should *not* do.

Don't cut your skin with a knife and try to suck out the venom like they did in the cowboy movies. You'll end up damaging your skin or severing nerves, arteries, or tendons in the process.

Don't think if there is only one fang mark on your skin that you haven't been bitten by a poisonous snake. I've seen several cases of poisonous snakebites with only one puncture wound. The poisonous snake you have encountered may be functioning with only one fang.

Don't put a cold compress on the wound or pack the wound in ice. Any skin tissue damaged by snake venom is highly sensitive to cold and will only feel worse. Icing the wound can also lead to superficial frostbite.

Don't apply a tourniquet to shut off the flow of arterial blood. Without proper training, most people apply a tourniquet too tightly and end up causing permanent damage to fingers or toes.

Don't bring a live snake to the Emergency Department. There have been cases where snakes have attacked doctors and patients right in the hospital. If you can safely kill the snake that bit you, show it to the doctor in order to identify it positively as a poisonous snake.

Don't panic. Fear stimulates the heart to pump faster, and this will only speed the venom more quickly into the body. Do your best to remain calm. Even with a severe poisoning, you have time to get to the hospital before symptoms worsen. However, the antidote must be administered no later than twelve hours after the attack in order to be effective.

Most snakebites are on the hands or arms. After being bitten, keep the arm immobilized with a splint. If possible, tie two twigs together to keep the arm from moving and hold it lower than the heart to slow the venom from reaching the heart. Otherwise, put the arm in a sling and hold it close to the body. If you are bitten on the leg, don't walk unless necessary. Again, this will lessen the possibilities of pumping the venom to the heart.

If you don't have anyone to take you to the Emergency Department for observation or treatment, call 911 or the EMS to get help at the scene or provide transportation.

Most poisonous snakebites, particularly those from rattlesnakes, are treated with special antivenom serum that is administered intravenously. For a minimal poisoning, you'll need three to five vials of serum. A major attack requires anywhere from twenty to thirty vials. The serum counteracts the snake poison, but will give flulike symptoms of aches and pains that can last for up to a month after the attack.

A nonpoisonous snake does not have fangs, only teeth. If bitten by a snake you are positive is nonpoisonous, clean the wound with soap and warm water.

Prevention

- Whenever you enter the habitat of a poisonous snake, wear long pants and high boots, especially when you go off the main trail.
- If you're going deep in the woods, far from the nearest hospital, take a snake-bite kit along and know how to use it properly.
- When hiking, don't stick your hands under rocks or in wood piles unless you are wearing thick leather gloves, or are certain no snakes are there.
- Carry a walking stick and bang on the ground as you go. If you make a racket, you won't surprise a snake, and it will have time to slither away.

What the Doctor Will Do

Contact your doctor if the wound from a nonpoisonous snake is particularly deep, or your tetanus shots are not up to date. Antibiotics may be prescribed as a precaution against bacterial infection.

WHAT TO DO

- Don't cut your skin with a knife to suck out the venom.
- Don't put a cold compress on the wound or pack it in ice.
- Don't apply a tourniquet in order to shut off the flow of arterial blood.
- Don't panic. Fear stimulates the heart to pump faster, and this will speed the flow of venom to the heart.

If you are bitten by a snake and are positive it is nonpoisonous:
- Clean the wound with soap and warm water.
- Contact your physician if the wound is deep, or your tetanus shots are not up to date.

SNORING

Aaron E. Sher, M.D.

Dr. Sher is clinical associate professor of surgery (Otolaryngology) and clinical associate professor of Pediatrics, Albany Medical College, and associate medical director for Sleep Related Breathing Disorders at Capital Region Sleep–Wake Disorder Center, Albany, New York

Millions of Americans snore, and the question is: Except for keeping someone awake at night, is snoring a problem? The answer is that it may or may not be.

Some snoring just means additional noise while sleeping. But chronic loud snoring may signify that the airways shut down periodically in the night, depriving the lungs of enough air. This is a serious medical problem called obstructive sleep apnea.

Snoring happens when the muscles that keep open the airways carrying air from the nose and throat to the lungs relax during sleep. This causes the airways to collapse, requiring more forceful inhalation to breathe.

Snoring can be brought on by enlarged tonsils and adenoids, nasal polyps, a tumor growing on the tongue, a deviated septum, an allergy or a bad cold, sleeping in an overly heated room, overconsumption of alcohol, sleeping pills, obesity, or in rare cases, a deformity of the craniofacial skeleton.

Snoring is predominantly a male adult ailment, but children between the ages of three and thirteen will snore when they have large tonsils and adenoids, or when they have a heavy cold. As they mature physically, most will naturally stop snoring.

Generally, adults start to snore in their late thirties and forties, and the incidences increase when men pass the age of fifty. Obesity can cause you to snore at any age.

Treatment

No one is certain why weight gain causes snoring, but it will. It may be linked to increased fat in the structures around the throat. This diminishes the size of the air passages through which you breathe. If you have a tendency to snore, it will get worse when you gain weight, and if you gain enough weight, you'll develop sleep apnea. If you already have mild sleep apnea, being overweight will worsen it. If you are overweight, begin to exercise on a regular basis in order to lose the excess weight.

Avoid all types of alcohol in the evening. Alcohol causes greater than normal relaxation of the throat muscles and will cause a nonsnorer to snore.

Do not take sleeping pills. The medication in many sleeping pills suppresses muscle tone just like alcohol.

Don't lie on your back because this position may lead to snoring. The best sleep positions are the stomach and side. However, for heavy snorers, sleep position has no effect; they will snore in all positions. To make sure that you sleep on your side, attach a sock with tennis balls inside it to the back of your sleepwear. When you roll over on your back in your sleep, the uncomfortable feeling will quickly cause you to return to your side.

Make sure there is a good flow of fresh air in the bedroom. When the room is hot and dry, nasal passages become clogged during sleep, and this often leads to snoring. If necessary, use a humidifier in the bedroom to keep the nasal passages moist when you sleep.

If you have allergies or nasal congestion due to a cold, this can restrict the air passages and cause snoring. Occasional use of a nasal decongestant before bedtime helps to keep the airways open while you sleep. However, chronic use of a decongestant is to be avoided except under medical advice and supervision.

If these self-help measures fail to stop you from snoring and if the snoring is regularly interfering with the sleep of your bed partner, or if you think that you may have obstructive sleep apnea, contact a sleep disorder center in your area.

The American Sleep Disorders Association (604 Second Street, S.W., Rochester, MN 55902; 507-287-6006) can provide nationwide referrals to sleep specialists—doctors trained in neurology, psychology, or pulmonary medicine—and also put you in touch with regional sleep centers in your area.

Cause for Concern

Sleep apnea is a potentially life-threatening disorder. Symptoms include loud snoring punctuated by quiet periods of a few seconds to 2 minutes where there is no breathing, followed again by a snort and loud snoring. Other signs of sleep apnea include chronic daytime fatigue, a morning headache, a sore throat, and dryness in the mouth in the morning following a night of breathing through the mouth.

Sleep apnea places a severe strain on the cardiovascular system and can lead to hypertension, nighttime heart attacks, cardiac arrhythmias, and stroke. It can also worsen asthma or existing cardiac disease. People with sleep apnea are typically obese, young to middle-aged males. The male to female ratio is 20–1, with practically all females postmenopausal.

What the Doctor Will Do

After a complete physical exam to rule out a physical obstruction, the doctor may recommend CPAP, or Continuous Positive Airway Pressure. This portable air pump and face mask is used every night to generate continuous air pressure through the nostrils and keep the throat from collapsing as you sleep. Both snoring and apnea are eliminated. One night of sleep with CPAP can have a major impact on people's lives when they see how it feels to wake up refreshed.

If other measures have failed, surgery to open the narrowed portions of the air passages may be required.

Even the most severe case of sleep apnea is curable by one or a combination of these approaches. In children with sleep apnea, removal of the tonsils and adenoids is often all that is required.

WHAT TO DO

- Lose excess weight.
- Do not take sleeping pills.
- Don't sleep on your back.

- Make sure there is a good flow of fresh air in the bedroom.
- Use a nasal humidifier to keep the nasal passages moist.
- Use a decongestant before bedtime if you have nasal congestion due to a cold.
- Seek treatment for allergies that cause nasal obstruction.

- If these measures fail to stop you from snoring, or if you think you may have obstructive sleep apnea, a potentially dangerous health risk typified by continuous nightly cycles of snoring and then no breathing at all, contact a sleep disorder center in your area.

STRESS

Col. Robert S. Brown, Ph.D., M.D.

Colonel Brown is clinical professor of behavioral medicine and psychiatry, professor of education, University of Virginia, and chief of Psychiatric Out-Patient Services, Kenner Army Hospital, Fort Lee, Virginia

Stress is caused by situations or circumstances—stressors—that threaten a person's mental or physical sense of well-being or feelings of balance. The more common stressors include family conflicts, marital discord or divorce, financial woe, deadlines, arguments or disagreements with others, conflicts at work, and the death of loved ones.

In almost every form of stress, the body prepares itself for the "fight or flight" response. Stress causes the release into the bloodstream of adrenaline and noradrenaline, two hormones that help you meet the perceived challenge. This leads to increased heart rate and elevated blood pressure, perspiration, muscle tension in the stomach or chest, headache, or feelings of hostility, fear, anxiety, or anger. Hyperventilation, which is typified by rapid and shallow breathing, can also occur.

This hormonal response is a throwback to early humans who needed the extra energy to fend off danger by attack or to track down a meal. This strong response is rarely needed anymore, but emotional distress from everyday living still triggers it.

Not all stress is negative. Sometimes a situation is presented as a challenge, a motivation to gather your forces and do your best. This positive stress makes life interesting and can give meaning and direction to your day.

Treatment

Whenever you feel stressed, make a conscious assessment of its sources. When you do this, you gain perspective and are able to decide how best to handle the stressor.

If you are unable to deal with the problem by yourself, find out who or what are the available resources that can help you. Contact a friend, an accountant, a minister, or a support group. Don't try to go it alone continually in the face of stress.

Symptoms of stress such as panic, anger, hostility, and fatigue have been traditionally treated in our society with tranquilizers, ulcer medication and antacids to relieve stomach distress, and sleeping aids to lull one to sleep. However, I find that stress is something we can usually control without medication. This takes a conscious and continual effort on your part.

When stress builds and the body is preparing to flee, then why not flee? Go and exercise to overcome the stress. Of course, if you're trapped in an office, or miss an appointment because of an airplane delay, you don't have access to physical release, and this can lead to pent-up frustration, anger, and misery. However, if your body is properly prepared through exercise, your resting heart rate and resting blood pressure will be lower than that of a sedentary person. When stress develops, a lower heart rate means a less severe reaction to stress. Also, the fitter you are, the quicker you should recover from the stress. Exercise seems to confer a sense of accomplishment and calm, and contributes to an overall sense of relaxation.

Another way to relieve stress is to talk with somebody about the situation. The first thing I do when I sense something disturbing is to call my wife. I go through the things that are bothering me, and together we try to arrive at a solution.

Talking to someone who wants to listen and understand is one of the most rewarding experiences of life. A loved one, a good friend—such as a family member, a family doctor, or a religious leader—can all be very helpful in this regard.

When stressed, I also think: Am I exaggerating the threat and minimizing my resources?

I go straight to my psychological reserve vault. This is an internal bank that's built on my positive daily body-mind-spirit experiences. Making use of these reserves in times of stress is just like going to the bank to withdraw a portion of your savings.

My physical reserve consists of my body and how well I take care of it. I jog five days a week, and follow my runs with a series of push-ups and sit-ups. I watch my diet and take no sleeping aids.

Rest and proper nutrition are also critical in fighting stress. Keep regular sleep hours. One of the major reasons people are stressed is because they are sleep-deprived. Their nerves are shot, and their response to stress is often negative. A poor diet also contributes to a negative response to stress. Take time for nourishing meals, just as an athlete does, to meet the special demands of stress.

The hallmark of personal responsibility is the ability to choose your responses to stress. You don't have to shout at someone who has offended you. Think things over before acting. Try to see where you or the other person is coming from. Elevate your thinking from the level of daily crisis management to the level of long-term management of your goals.

I have a spiritual side. This adds value and meaning to my life. Whether you believe in God or not, whether you are religious or not, it is the spiritual side, exemplified by kindness and courtesy toward others, that produces feelings of well-being. These feelings are important and help you to put life's events in better perspective. Go out of your way to help somebody, and you will find that it can work wonders toward stress relief.

When these variables are deposited in my bank each day, there is almost no stress that can overwhelm me. Whenever I have depleted my reserve because of inattention or overwork, I become irritated, don't cope well, and become easily angered and frustrated.

The real secret to stress management is learning how to get along with other people. Be flexible enough in your ideas and attitudes to listen to others and be able to shift your ideas when needed. Be oriented toward the needs of others, and it is amazing how much easier things will become.

If you live alone, or if you spend a great deal of time by yourself, a pet can be a valuable asset. Research has shown people feel better and live longer if they have someone or something to take care of. A pet, whether it be a cat, a dog, or a bird, can play an important role in your life.

There is nothing more important than the psychological environment that we create for ourselves. So, when I get up in the morning I put a classical music station on the radio. The music helps provide me with relaxation, inspiration, distraction, and meaning. Listen to whatever type of music relaxes you. Choose a quiet room with no distractions and turn the music on. Focus on the melody or words, and use the music to help calm yourself.

What the Doctor Will Do

If you try dealing with stress but continue to suffer from it, contact your family physician for help. There is nothing more valuable than a caring doctor. The doctor may be able to provide other solutions to your problems.

A psychiatrist may be recommended for further evaluation. If medication is needed, it may be for a short term as you work together to find a long-term cure.

WHAT TO DO

- Learn to change your reactions to stressors and neutralize them so you don't become angry, humiliated, sad, ill, or unduly anxious.
- Find out who or what the available resources are that can help you if you are unable to deal with the problem by yourself.
- Exercise regularly to calm down and help overcome stress. Walking or other simple exercises are highly beneficial.
- Talk to someone who wants to listen and understand and also share his or her thoughts with you.
- Avoid denial or minimizing a situation that is bothering you.
- Keep regular sleep hours.
- Take time for nourishing meals.
- Have appropriate medical exams and seek medical attention when you have an illness.
- Think things over before reacting to a stressor.
- Go out of your way to help someone. Sharing and caring toward your neighbor works wonders for stress relief.
- Be flexible in your ideas and attitudes; willing to change your perceptions when indicated.
- Listen to music that relaxes you and helps lessen feelings of stress.
- If you still suffer from stress, contact your family physician for help. If the doctor can't provide solutions for your problems, a psychiatrist may be recommended for further evaluation.

VARICOSE VEINS

Julius H. Jacobson II, M.D.

*Dr. Jacobson is professor of surgery, Mount Sinai School of Medicine,
and director, vascular surgery, Mount Sinai Hospital in New York City*

Varicose veins, the swollen, oftentimes tender leg veins near the skin surface, can bring on feelings of heaviness, fatigue, itching, and scaling of the legs. They now affect over 80 million Americans, and typically appear at the back of the calf or anywhere on the length of the inside part of the leg. In most cases, varicose veins ache after you walk even a short distance, or after standing for prolonged periods. Fortunately, they are usually benign, more of a cosmetic than a medical concern.

There are many causes of varicose veins, and there is no proof that genetics plays a role. It's estimated that 40 percent of all women have varicose veins, in most cases caused by childbearing. The weight of a fetus during pregnancy places stress on the leg veins and causes them to dilate. In addition, during pregnancy certain hormones are released that relax the veins and cause them to become bigger. Birth-control pills can also increase your risk for varicose veins as well as phlebitis, an inflammation of the wall of a vein. This can lead to more varicose veins because of the increased valve destruction.

Obesity is also a common cause of varicose veins because excess weight, combined with a reduction in activity, leads to more pressure on the leg veins.

Age is another cause. As you get older, veins lose their natural elasticity and become more susceptible to damage.

A sedentary life-style can result in varicose veins since inactivity causes blood to collect in the veins of the legs, leading to excessive pressure and subsequent vein damage.

Prevention

Several things can reduce your chances of developing varicose veins or, if you already have some, minimize their effects:

- Walk regularly in order to keep your calf pump in good working order.
- Exercise regularly and vigorously. Running, bicycling, swimming, dancing, and cross-country skiing are some activities that will improve overall circulation, help control weight, and keep blood from pooling in the legs.
- Don't stand still or sit for prolonged periods of time. If you are riding on a plane, keep your heels on the floor and gently raise your toes up and down twenty times. Repeat this every hour.
- If your job demands you be immobile for extended periods, do simple toe raises every now and then to get the calf muscles pumping blood back to the heart. To perform a toe raise, stand flat-footed, then rise up onto the balls of your feet, hold that position momentarily, and then go back down to the floor. Repeat this twenty times.
- If you sit for a long time, get up and walk for several minutes. Keep your legs raised whenever possible to aid blood flow back to the heart. Sleep with your feet propped up on a pillow.

- When sitting, don't cross your legs at the knee. This creates pressure on the leg veins.
- Don't wear tight pantyhose or girdles. They compress and restrict the veins around the thighs and make it hard for blood to move upward.

Treatment

If you are concerned about the appearance of your varicose veins, or if they cause your foot and ankle to swell, you have two options.

The first is to wear special support stockings, which can improve circulation somewhat but won't cure your condition. The stockings are available at surgical supply houses or can be custom-fitted for you, usually at the same store. They come in knee, full-length, or panty hose—prescribed according to the severity of the varicose veins—and are put on in the morning before your feet touch the floor and taken off at night before going to bed.

The second option is surgery, which is described below.

What the Doctor Will Do

If I had varicose veins and was upset at how they looked, I would have them surgically removed with a basic procedure called vein stripping. I'd rather spend a day at the hospital than put on tight stockings for the rest of my life.

In its simplest form, the surgeon makes a small incision at the groin and another small incision at the ankle. A special instrument is passed up that hooks onto the affected veins and pulls them out. Blood from the damaged veins then flows to veins with good valves. The leg is wrapped tightly in an elastic bandage to prevent bleeding, and it's kept on for a week. If the half-hour surgery is performed on a Friday, you can go back to work on the following Monday in many cases. Extensive walking is a big part of the recovery process.

A highly publicized alternative method to traditional surgery is called sclerotherapy, in which a chemical is injected into the damaged veins. I don't believe in this procedure at all, especially when it's used for the treatment of tiny red varicose veins called "spider veins." If you find spider veins to be offensive, the best way to deal with them is with special cover-up make-up available at any pharmacy or department store.

The total cost in time and money for sclerotherapy is much more than vein stripping procedures performed at hospitals. Then, too, many of the doctors performing this nonsurgical procedure out of their offices or in special "vein clinics" are unethical, incompetent quacks. Many abuses have already been reported to medical authorities.

Cause for Concern

If you develop any redness or tenderness, or notice a distinct swelling along the length of a varicose vein in your leg, contact your physician. You may have superficial phlebitis, a vein inflammation usually caused by an infection. Prescription medication, hot compresses, and an elastic support bandage will generally take care of this in a matter of weeks.

WHAT TO DO

- Wear special support stockings to keep the veins collapsed and prevent them from increasing in size.
- Walk regularly in order to keep the leg muscles pumping blood back to the heart.
- Exercise regularly and vigorously to improve overall circulation, control weight, and keep blood from pooling in the legs.
- Do simple toe raises to improve leg circulation.
- Don't cross your legs at the knees.
- Don't wear tight pantyhose or girdles.
- If you are concerned about the appearance of your varicose veins, or if they cause your foot and ankle to swell, or if they become red, tender, or swollen along the length of a varicose vein, contact your physician.

Appendices

MEDICAL EMERGENCY

E. Jackson Allison, Jr., M.D., M.P.H., F.A.C.E.P.

Dr. Allison is president of the American College of Emergency Physicians, and Sterling Distinguished Professor and Chair of the Department of Emergency Medicine at East Carolina University School of Medicine in Greenville, North Carolina

Common illnesses and injuries often require immediate medical attention. When your family physician isn't available, or if the illness or injury is traumatic, go directly to the hospital Emergency Department for diagnosis and treatment. Better still, call 911 and get there by ambulance. You'll get attended to quicker.

There are over 5,000 Emergency Departments in hospitals throughout the country, and most are full-service facilities with trained emergency personnel in attendance around the clock.

Many people have the misconception that "emergency rooms" are mainly for cardiac cases. Not so. Today these are full-fledged Emergency Departments, actually minihospitals with all the equipment and staff to treat every type of medical and dental emergency. At my hospital we treat over 47,000 people a year, with cases ranging from spider bites to compound fractures, earaches, vaginal bleeding, car crashes, poisoning, diarrhea, bullet wounds, lacerations, and heart attacks.

Be prepared for medical emergencies. If you live in a region that has several Emergency Departments within easy travel, find the one that best suits your needs. An important factor in this decision is the reputation of each facility. If an Emergency Department is well-regarded in your community, then one can feel more confident in seeking out its services in time of need.

Another important factor is location. Take a trip to the hospital and see how long it takes. Find out the best route to follow. Once at the hospital, find where the Emergency Department is located and where you can park your car.

In some medical emergencies you will have no choice but to go to the nearest hospital Emergency Department for treatment. If hospitalization is required, arrangements can be made to be transferred to the hospital of your choice.

Medical Emergency Warning Signs

Emergency treatment is needed for the following reasons:

- Unconsciousness.
- Fainting followed by numbness, confusion, difficulty speaking, or blurred vision.
- Pain or pressure in the chest and upper abdominal area.
- Slurring of words.
- Shortness of breath, difficulty breathing.
- Bullet or stab wounds.
- Broken bones.
- Head injury.
- Eye damage.
- Poisoning.
- Smoke or noxious fume inhalation.
- Uncontrollable bleeding.
- Dehydration.
- Prolonged vomiting or diarrhea.
- Drug overdose.
- Snake, animal, or insect bites.
- Frostbite.

The Emergency Department

Depending on the severity of the complaint, you can either drive yourself, have a friend or family member take you, or call for an ambulance. *For any severe chest pain lasting 2 minutes or more, or if the pain spreads to the shoulders, jaw, neck or arms, call for an ambulance.* You may be experiencing a heart attack and may need immediate medical attention.

When you call 911 for help, speak calmly and clearly, giving the nature of the problem and providing the name, address, phone number, and location of the victim. Don't hang up until the dispatcher has all the information.

Once you arrive at the Emergency Department, triage, or sorting, begins in order to see who is in need of immediate attention. Federal and state law(s) allow treatment in Emergency Departments regardless of insurance coverage or ability to pay, so the staff won't perform a "wallet biopsy" before they begin. However, it would be helpful to bring along any insurance information that you may have.

There are three broad triage categories used in the Emergency Department, and treatment is administered according to critical need, not on a first-come, first-served basis. As you wait, ambulances will often bring in critical-care patients through other entrances, so your treatment may be delayed if you don't have a life- or limb-threatening problem.

Triage categories are differentiated as follows:

Category 1. Needs immediate attention. Chest pain, vital signs are unstable, ashen appearance, perspiring. "FTD" (Fixin' to Die) appearance. This also includes severe head trauma and other similar cases.

Category 2. Needs attention soon. Noncomplicated fracture, stable vital signs.

Category 3. Nonemergency. The least ill, but wants or may need an exam for a self-limiting illness. No matter what the doctor does, the patient will get better in time.

How to Prevent Medical Emergencies

Prevention is the best remedy. In order to prevent many of the all too common accidents that occur in and around the home, be sure to do the following:

- Cover all electrical sockets if you have very young children in the home.
- Store all pots and pans and other non-dangerous items on low shelves in the kitchen and move all chemicals up high out of the reach of children.
- Keep all toys and clothing off the stairs to prevent falls.
- Keep all medications out of the reach of children. Use child-resistant caps.
- Keep syrup of ipecac in the home in case of poisoning.
- Keep the number of the local poison control center near your phone.
- Be ever-vigilant for people in the home less able to take care of themselves.

The First-Aid Kit

Keep a complete first-aid kit in the home. Be sure that the following items are included in it:

- Adhesive bandages in a variety of sizes, including butterfly bandages, for taking care of scrapes, cuts, and wounds.
- Gauze pads in 2- and 4-inch sizes to dress cuts and puncture wounds.
- Antibiotic ointment for cuts and scrapes.
- Instant activating ice bags for cold applications for sprains and possible fracture(s).
- Tape.
- Scissors.
- Triangular cloth for arm sling.
- Aspirin, acetaminophen, or ibuprofen for pain, fever, and headache.
- Elastic wrap for supporting and compressing injuries to the knee, ankle, elbow, and wrist.
- Syrup of ipecac to induce vomiting.
- Thermometer.
- Prescription insect bite kit or food allergy kit if you have known allergies to bees, wasps, or certain foods.

READING YOUR PRESCRIPTION

Steven Lamm, M.D.

Dr. Lamm is assistant clinical professor of medicine,
New York University School of Medicine in New York City

Making sense of a doctor's written prescription can be difficult. A doctor's handwriting is often a seemingly unintelligible scrawl, not to mention the mysterious series of Latin abbreviations that specify how the chemist or pharmacist should fill the prescription. (Occasionally, as a result of poor handwriting, you may receive the wrong medication or dosage. If you develop unusual side effects after taking the medication, call your doctor immediately.)

Narcotics are usually prescribed on a different type of prescription form (this may vary from state to state) and written in triplicate in order to better control the dispensing of the drugs.

When the patent runs out on a prescription medication, other pharmaceutical companies may then manufacture the medication in equal biologic potency. This is called a generic drug. These generic drugs will probably cost less than the nongeneric equivalent.

At times, even though a generic drug may be available, for a variety of reasons your physician may elect to prescribe the brand medication instead. The physician may feel that the generic drug is not equivalent. Or the doctor may want you to take the same colored pill every day to eliminate any risk of confusion over which pill to take. This can be important with elderly people who often take a variety of daily medications.

With certain drugs, it is important to maintain a certain level in the system for efficacy. This occurs with hormone medications, blood thinners, and psychotropic drugs. The doctor may want you to take the same brand with each prescription refill and would write "daw" on the prescription form.

Understanding a few of these frequently used terms the doctor writes on the prescription form will help take some of the mystique out of medications and give you a greater sense of your own health.

When I write a prescription, these are some of the commonly used abbreviations, many in Latin, and their meanings:
- ac: before meals
- bid: twice daily
- c: with
- daw: dispense as written, nongeneric form of drug
- gtt: drops
- hs: at bedtime
- non rep: no refill
- pc: after meals
- po: by mouth
- prn: as needed
- qh: every hour
- qid: four times daily
- rep: refill
- s: without
- Sig: directions
- tid: three times daily

DIRECTORY OF NATIONAL HEALTH ORGANIZATIONS

The following resources provide basic information about various diseases, illnesses, and medical problems. Some have written information free for the asking or for a nominal fee. In many cases, the groups will provide names of physicians, health specialists, and other resources available in your region to assist you further with your medical queries.

ASTHMA
(800) 222-LUNG
National Jewish Hospital/National
Asthma Center

HEALTH INFORMATION
(800) 336-4797
Provides referrals to national
organizations dealing with various
illnesses.

Centers for Disease Control
Department of Health and Human
  Services
Public Inquiries
Building 1, Room B63
1600 Clifton Road, N.E.
Atlanta, Georgia 30333
(404) 329-3534

Office of Consumer and Professional
  Affairs
Food and Drug Administration, HFN17
5600 Fishers Lane
Rockville, Maryland 20857
(301) 295-8012
Answers questions about safety of
  medications.

Arthritis Foundation
1314 Spring Street N.W.
Atlanta, Georgia 30309
(404) 872-7100

National Women's Health Network
224 7th Street S.E.
Washington, D.C. 20003
(202) 543-9222

Skin Cancer Foundation
475 Park Avenue South
New York, New York 10016
(212) 725-5176

National Migraine Foundation
5252 N. Western Avenue
Chicago, Illinois 66025
(312) 878-7715

American Osteopathic Association
212 E. Ohio Avenue
Chicago, Illinois 60611
(312) 280-5882
Refers to osteopathic hospitals and
  osteopaths in your area.

The National Psoriasis Foundation
Suite 210
6443 S.W. Beaverton Highway
Portland, Oregon 97221
(503) 297-1545
Clearinghouse for information about
  psoriasis.

American Academy of Allergy and
  Immunology
611 E. Wells Street
Milwaukee, Wisconsin 53202
(414) 272-6071

American Lung Association
1740 Broadway
New York, New York 10019
(212) 315-8700

American Medical Association
535 North Dearborn Street
Chicago, Illinois 60610
(312) 645-5000

Index

mouth (cont.)
    see also tooth and mouth
        problems
mouthwashes, 101
mucus:
    blood in, 119
    loosening of, 118
muscle and joint problems:
    arthritis, 66, 68–71, 72, 73, 91,
        146–47, 152, 202, 229, 230
    carpal tunnel syndrome, 66, 72–
        73
    common, 66–67
    dislocations, 67–68
    emergencies, 67–68
    fractures, 68, 85, 86, 153
    ganglions, 68
    hammertoe, 68
    lower back pain, 66, 73–78
    muscle cramps, 66, 83–85
    muscle soreness or pain, 66, 78–
        82, 116
    osteoporosis, 68
    requiring physician's care, 68
    shin splints, 66, 85–87
    sprains, 66, 87–90
    stiff neck, 67, 90–94, 221
    tendinitis, 67, 94–96
muscle cramps, 66, 83–85
    causes for concern with, 84
    prevention of, 83
    treatment of, 84
    what to do for, 84–85
muscles and joints, 65–96
    flexibility of, 80
    general information on, 65–68
    mini stretching and
        strengthening program for,
        80–82
    specialists for, 65–67
muscle soreness and pain, 66, 78–
    82
    causes for concern in, 82
    colds and, 116
    doctor's care of, 82
    mini stretching and
        strengthening program for,
        80–82
    prevention of, 80
    treatment of, 79–80
    what to do for, 82
musculoskeletal specialists, 65–67
music, in stress management, 240
Mycelex, 145
Mycolog, 189
Mylanta II, 50

Mylicon, 50
myopia, flashes and, 19
myringotomy, 31

nails, see fingernails; toenails
napping:
    insomnia and, 225
    jet lag and, 228
Naprosyn, 134
naproxen, 134
narcotics, 247
nasal congestion:
    colds and, 115–16, 129
    snoring and, 238
nasal decongestants, 116, 237
    for airplane ears, 28
    sprays, 28, 125, 129
national health organizations, 248–
    249
National Migraine Foundation,
    249
National Psoriasis Foundation, 249
National Women's Health
    Network, 249
nausea, 40, 61–64
    causes for concern with, 63–64
    food poisoning and, 51, 61, 62
    treatment of, 62–63
    what to do for, 64
nearsightedness, flashes and, 19
neck:
    stiff, 67, 90–94, 221
    strengthening exercises for, 92–
        93
    stretching exercises for, 92
Neosporin, 178, 181
nerve root impingement, 90–91
neuromas, 156
Neutrogena hand cream, 181
nickel, allergies to, 188
nicotine, 211, 216, 226
    see also smoking
nightclothes, 139
911 calls, 245, 246
nitrites, 222
Nix, 198
nocturnal cramping, 83
noise, sleep disrupted by, 224
noradrenaline, 238
nose, 112
    congested, see nasal congestion
nosebleeds, 231–33
    causes for concern with, 232
    causes of, 231
    prevention of, 232
    treatment of, 231–32

what the doctor will do for, 233
what to do for, 233
nylon, 217

oatmeal treatments:
    for hives, 191
    for itch relief, 187
    for psoriasis, 202
obesity and overweight:
    cervical spine degeneration and,
        91–92
    collapsed arches and, 158
    heartburn and, 54, 55
    heel pain and, 152
    jock itch and, 196
    lower back pain and, 74
    psoriasis and, 202
    snoring and, 236
    sore feet and, 156
    stasis eczema and, 189
    stiff neck and, 90
    urinary stress incontinence and,
        141
    varicose veins and, 241
obstetricians, 133
odor, foot, 143, 150–51
Office of Consumer and
    Professional Affairs, 249
oil glands:
    aging and, 211
    boils and, 168
    inflammation of (acne), 164–
        166
ointments:
    burns worsened by, 173
    see also antibiotic creams and
        ointments
open comedos (blackheads), 164,
    165
ophthalmologists, 14
opossums, 214
opticians, 14
optic nerve, 12
optometrists, 14
Orabase, 178
oral contraceptives, see birth
    control pills
oral hygiene, 97, 101
oral pathologists, 98, 104
oral surgeons, 97
orbits (eye sockets), 12
    blowout fractures of, 15
orthodontists, 98
orthopedic emergencies, 67–68
orthopedic problems, see muscle
    and joint problems